SMQs

DEVELOPMENT AND RATIONAL USE OF STANDARDISED MedDRA QUERIES (SMQs)

Retrieving Adverse Drug Reactions with MedDRA

Report of the CIOMS Working Group

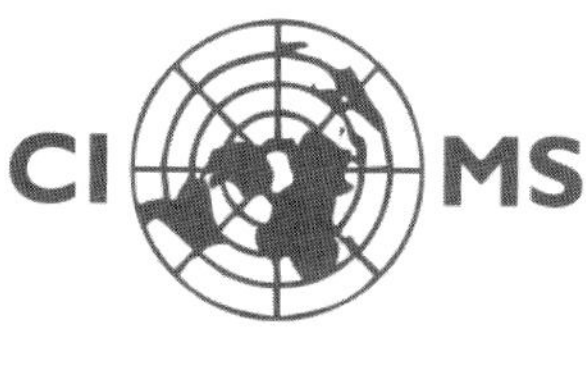

Geneva 2004

ISBN 92 9036 077 1
Printed in Switzerland

TABLE OF CONTENTS

I. INTRODUCTION

During its many years of existence, one of the roles of CIOMS has been to take up contentious research ethics issues as well as issues related to drug safety and drug development research and help to resolve them through specially organized working groups comprised of representatives of all the interested parties as stakeholders. This role of serving as a neutral platform for the public and private sectors as well as for the scientific community has proved its utility on many occasions in the past. A similar approach was also initially considered in the case of this undertaking.

Historically, the project with practical suggestions described in this publication began as a CIOMS initiative, in response to indications received from some drug regulatory authorities and pharmaceutical companies that they had concerns about the parallel development of special drug safety search programmes based on the Medical Dictionary for Regulatory Activities (MedDRA). This would cause an unavoidable duplication of effort and uncertainty within the pharmaceutical companies about the utility of these searches on the part of drug regulatory authorities.

MedDRA has been developed by the International Conference on Harmonisation (ICH) and is being implemented worldwide by drug regulatory authorities, the pharmaceutical and biotechnology industry, and academia for coding, reporting, analysing, and communicating regulatory and drug safety information. The size and complexity of MedDRA terminology carries the risk that different users may select differing sets of terms while trying to retrieve cases relative to the same drug safety problem. It has also been stressed that the active participation of drug regulatory authorities in the preparation of search queries is essential for their subsequent acceptance of search results and that there is a need to agree upon how the search results should be presented using a specially designed template.

A CIOMS Working Group on the Rational Use of MedDRA Terminology for Drug Safety Database Searches was established in May 2002. The original 24 members were senior scientists representing seven drug regulatory authorities, seven pharmaceutical companies, as well as other organizations such as WHO. Initially, it had been planned to proceed by consensus of the Working Group members, along the concept of a "users' group", i.e. without the direct involvement of the MedDRA Maintenance and Support Services Organization (MSSO), by selecting from the MedDRA sets of terms which met specific search criteria and retrieval problems. The aim was to publish them in a medical journal, and offer them for general use, in line with earlier CIOMS projects such as "Reporting Adverse Drug Reactions: Definitions of Terms and Criteria for Their Use" (CIOMS, Geneva, 1999, ISBN 92 9036 071 2). However, at an early stage it became clear that such an activity would benefit from cooperation between all stakeholders, i.e. between the CIOMS Working Group, the MedDRA Maintenance and Support Service Organisation (MedDRA MSSO), the ICH MedDRA Management Board and the ICH Secretariat. This was particularly so as MSSO also recognised that MedDRA's special Search Categories did not meet the user communities general data retrieval needs and had started to develop a new tool – MedDRA Analytical Groupings (MAGs) intended to serve similar objectives. This collaborative effort was designed to take full advantage of expertise, technical capabilities, administrative procedures, other ongoing harmonisation activities, maintenance of search queries, etc. In May 2003, the Working Group was renamed the CIOMS Working Group on Standardised MedDRA Queries (SMQs).

Traditionally, the results of all CIOMS activities, such as publications from working groups, guidelines, etc., have always been available without restriction to the entire scientific community, as opposed to the MedDRA documents, many of which are available only to subscribers. The aim of this CIOMS publication is to brief drug regulatory authorities, scientific institutions and pharmaceutical companies worldwide about the development, purpose and appropriate use of SMQs in drug surveillance. Two papers in this publication ("Application of Standardised MedDRA Queries (SMQs) in Pharmacovigilance" and "Template Concerning Communication of Search Results") are to assist in the rational use of search queries in the identification and retrieval of potentially relevant individual case safety reports from a database and to harmonise presentation of search results. The publication includes three candidate Standardised MedDRA Queries (SMQs) developed by the Working Group, namely *Torsade de Pointes*/QT Prolongation, Rhabdomyolysis/Myopathy and Hepatic disorders. It should be stressed that they are published only as examples to illustrate the structure and content of the end product, i.e. SMQs, but are by no means to be incorporated into any system or used routinely as search queries.

In parallel to this publication, the CIOMS Working Group on Standardised MedDRA Queries is continuing to work on the development of additional candidate SMQs. The progress made can be followed on the CIOMS website: www.cioms.ch/ What's New. In addition, for current information about the SMQ posting schedule, documents, etc., the MSSO website: www.meddramsso.com may also be consulted.

CIOMS would like to take this opportunity to thank all concerned for their valuable contributions and looks forward to their continued collaboration in the future.

Geneva, August 2004

Juhana E. Idänpään-Heikkilä, MD, PhD,
Secretary-General, CIOMS

Jan Venulet, MD,
Senior Adviser, CIOMS

II. Overview of Development Concepts Proposed by the Working Group

1. Executive Summary

The ICH process is being used by a Working Group to develop Standardised MedDRA Queries (SMQs). The Working Group, formed under the auspices of the Council for International Organizations of Medical Sciences (CIOMS), has representation from the three ICH Regions and the MedDRA Maintenance and Support Services Organization (MSSO); an ICH MedDRA Advisory Panel on SMQs provides oversight. SMQs are intended to aid in the identification and retrieval of potentially relevant individual case safety reports; SMQs are groupings of MedDRA terms, ordinarily at the Preferred Term (PT) level, that relate to a defined medical condition or area of interest. Terms included in a given SMQ may relate to relevant signs, symptoms, diagnoses, syndromes, physical findings, laboratory and other physiologic test data, etc. However, the methods used for SMQ development systematically exclude other parameters, such as timing of occurrence of an adverse event relative to drug administration, patient age, patient sex, disease severity, drug names, or case outcome. These other features may be essential elements of a given safety database search or an analysis of causality, but generally need to be considered separately from the adverse events of interest. The Working Group recommends that these adjunctive factors be considered, as indicated by the specific circumstances of the query, before or after the application of SMQs in the analytical sequence.

SMQs are not necessarily comprehensive, error-free, or universally applicable. However, results of performing a given SMQ search on a database should be reproducible and an identical search may be performed on any database utilizing the appropriate version of MedDRA. Thus, the overarching rationale for SMQs is to provide a framework for reproducible searches and to avoid expensive duplication of effort. SMQs are not intended to provide a final answer to a regulatory question(s), but rather provide a Standardised frame of reference for application when appropriate.

Development of SMQs is an interactive process, with many dependencies, and requires a cooperative consensus approach amongst all parties.

The Working Group is responsible for identifying medical conditions of interest, creating groupings of MedDRA terms for each Candidate SMQ, conducting pre-release testing on MedDRA-coded database(s), and developing guidance on when and how to use each SMQ. The Working Group modifies each Candidate SMQ based on results of testing and other feedback. As part of pre-release development, each Candidate SMQ undergoes testing with production data to reduce uncertainty about the utility of these searches. The MedDRA MSSO is responsible for defining the file structure to support the medical concepts behind each Candidate SMQ. In addition, the MSSO will make each Candidate SMQ available to all MedDRA subscribers for broader field testing and comment before formal release of the SMQ. The ICH MedDRA Advisory Panel on SMQs will advise the MedDRA Management Board concerning the status of SMQ development prior to formal acceptance by the Management Board and release of each SMQ by the MSSO. After launch, SMQs will be maintained by the MSSO to ensure compliance with the latest version of MedDRA; the MSSO will involve appropriate experts, when appropriate, to assess the potential impact of maintenance activities on the clinical relevance of each SMQ(s).

2. Background

MedDRA is a comprehensive and complex medical terminology developed by ICH that is being implemented worldwide by drug regulatory authorities, the pharmaceutical and biotechnology industry, and academia for coding, reporting, analyzing, and communicating regulatory information. MedDRA is especially useful for classification of drug safety information, but safety monitoring activities using data coded with MedDRA are particularly challenging due to the granularity of MedDRA. Identification of case reports with defined medical conditions or other areas of medical interest is a critical need for both Industry and Regulators.

To develop a Standardised approach to the identification of reports that represent, or could represent, important medical conditions with potential impact on benefit-risk evaluations, senior scientists from nine drug regulatory authorities, along with senior scientists from fourteen pharmaceutical companies, established a collaborative Working Group in cooperation with CIOMS. In addition, senior scientists from other organizations have contributed to the Working Group effort. See Table 1 for details.

Table 1. Participants in the CIOMS Working Group on Standardised MedDRA Queries (as at August 2004).

Regulatory Authorities:	Afssaps (France); BfArM[1] (Germany); EMEA[1] (European Union); FDA[1] (USA); Health Canada[1]; MHLW (Japan); MHRA[1] (United Kingdom); MPA[1] (Sweden); and TGA Australia
Pharmaceutical Industry:	AstraZeneca; Aventis[1]; Boehringer-Ingelheim[1]; Eisai; GlaxoSmithKline; Johnson and Johnson; Lilly; Novartis[1]; Organon; Pfizer[1]; Pharmacia[1]; Roche[1]; Schering AG (Germany) and Schering-Plough[1]
Others:	CIOMS Secretariat, Degge Group, Ltd.; Elliot Brown Consulting, Ltd.[1,2]; IFPMA (ICH Secretariat); MedDRA MSSO and JMO, and WHO[1] (Uppsala Monitoring Centre)

Notes: [1] Original Participant in the Working Group
[2] Resigned December 2003

The Working Group has adopted an open approach to SMQ development and input from all MedDRA stakeholders is encouraged. Any stakeholder may submit suggestions for new SMQ development, as well as provide feedback at any time during the development process or after final release of an SMQ. Stakeholders may direct comments to either the CIOMS Working Group or the MSSO. However, production release requests related to general maintenance of SMQs should be directed to the MSSO.

3. Definitions

Standardised MedDRA Queries (SMQs), which must be endorsed by the MedDRA Management Board prior to official release for use by subscribers, are groupings of MedDRA terms from one or more SOCs that relate to a defined medical condition or area of interest. They are intended to aid in identification and retrieval of potentially relevant reports from a drug safety database. The terms included may relate to signs, symptoms, diagnoses, syndromes, physical findings, laboratory and other physiologic test data, etc., that are associated with the medical condition or area of interest. SMQs include Preferred Term (PT) level terms, which represent unique medical concepts. However, SMQs may also include other levels of the MedDRA hierarchy. Relevant Lowest Level Terms (LLTs) are ordinarily included at the PT level; if a High Level Term (HLT) is included in a given SMQ, the HLT would ordinarily be represented in the SMQ by the entire set of PT level terms included under that HLT.

Candidate SMQs are preliminary descriptions of MedDRA search criteria and associated draft documentation, which must be agreed to by the Working Group before start of pre-release testing as described below. Ideally, the medical literature and/or medical specialists familiar with MedDRA terminology will be consulted on an ad hoc basis to review each Candidate SMQ for clinical relevance before pre-release testing.

See additional definitions, below, as applied to SMQ development.

4. ICH MedDRA Advisory Panel on SMQs

The main function of the ICH MedDRA Advisory Panel on SMQs, whose membership is designated by the six ICH Parties plus the UK MHRA and Health Canada, will be to give advice to the MedDRA Management Board concerning the development of MedDRA SMQs (including recommendation for the official endorsement of SMQs). The proposed duration of this Advisory Panel is for two years (starting from execution of the Memorandum of Understanding), with possible extension based on an assessment of the situation at that time.

5. General Applications of SMQs to Database Query

In the context of SMQ development, database queries refer to the searching of a drug safety database for individual reports that include adverse events relevant to a specified medical condition or other area of interest. SMQs are developed for identification and retrieval of case reports that are potentially relevant to a specific medical condition or other area of interest. Factors determining the search are principally medical in nature, but other parameters, such as timing of occurrence of an adverse event relative to drug administration, patient age, patient sex, disease severity, drug names, or case outcome, may be essential elements of any given safety database search or an analysis of causality. These are not aspects of database query that are covered by the present concept of SMQs. The Working Group recommends that these adjunctive factors be considered, as indicated by the specific circumstances of the query, before or after the application of SMQs in the analytical sequence.

In general, safety database queries, as outlined above, provide answers to one or both of these questions:

1) How many reports of a particular adverse event (or condition) described in MedDRA terms are represented in the database?
2) Which are the individual reports?

The Working Group recognizes that many factors can affect the results of database queries. Three critical factors are:

1) The extent to which the person performing the query understands medical terminology, medical conditions, and MedDRA;
2) The way the organization (i.e., database owner) has chose to implement MedDRA, including migration of legacy data from another terminology to MedDRA, versioning, and term selection and coding conventions for new data entry; and
3) The structure of the safety database, including the levels of MedDRA that can be accommodated and their linkages, as well as availability of search and output software, and whether features and functionality are available to fully utilize the multiaxiality of MedDRA.

Thus, as a practical matter, one of two general methods is used to construct a database query for identification and retrieval of individual case safety reports from a drug safety database:

1) A customized query can be created for the particular medicine and database under review; the search parameters are provided by known coded terms in the database at a certain point in time;
2) A query can be based on the entire medical terminology used for coding terms across many databases; search parameters are independent of the database and the query can be applied to any database using this terminology.

SMQs utilize the second approach, and take account of the scope and structure of MedDRA, i.e., search parameters are considered independent of the database so that the query will have applicability to any MedDRA-coded database. This approach takes advantage of the granularity of MedDRA and also provides an accommodation for slight differences in structured data that result from variation in coding conventions used for different databases.

As indicated above, certain factors, such as disease severity, drug names, and patient demographics that are not usually integral to MedDRA-coded data are excluded from SMQs unless, by exception, relevant terms are present in MedDRA. Because SMQs are based on MedDRA terms, their content is dependent upon the version of MedDRA used. This is specified for each search and it is necessary for the MSSO to ascertain whether version-related changes have occurred that will require modification to the SMQ search parameters in subsequent MedDRA versions. During the process of maintaining MedDRA and the SMQs, the MSSO will update each SMQ, producing an equivalent SMQ (version) for each MedDRA version. If the database in use does not contain the same version of MedDRA stipulated for the search, results may be different from that intended by the Working Group. Thus, it is important for the user to select the correct version of the SMQ for the MedDRA version in the subject database. Additional potential limitations are described in a separate section, below.

As each SMQ is developed, the Working Group creates guidance on when and how to use the respective SMQ. In addition, the Working Group makes recommendations on reporting results of SMQs in the spirit of transparency.

6. Development of Candidate SMQs

Specific medical conditions were selected for SMQ development by a consensus process and prioritized for development by the CIOMS Working Group. Working Group members contributed suggestions based on their pharmacovigilance experience and the MSSO provided additional suggestions based on work with MedDRA Analytical Groupings. Detail of the method used by the Working Group to prepare each Candidate SMQ is provided with each SMQ. However, a general description of the approach is as follows: Once the key medical concepts that are relevant to the condition under consideration have been identified and agreed upon, an SMQ team from the Working Group constructs groupings of MedDRA terms for the Candidate SMQ by searching the MedDRA hierarchy. First, a series of "bottom up" searches of MedDRA is conducted across all SOCs to locate key terms at the LLT level that are relevant to the medical concepts of interest. This is followed by identification of the PTs associated with the identified LLTs and their superordinate group terms (HLTs, HLGTs, and SOCs). Then a focused "top down" review of the MedDRA hierarchy is carried out to identify additional relevant PTs under the group terms that were initially not identified in the "bottom up" search. By using this combination of strategies, it is expected that this approach will yield most, if not all, of the relevant and appropriate MedDRA terms for the Candidate SMQ.

The MSSO will create the file format required to support each SMQ and this will be described in user guidance documents that complement each SMQ.

7. Rationale for Selection of Terms

SMQs may have a mixture of very specific terms and less specific terms that are consistent with a description of the overall clinical syndrome associated with a particular adverse event and drug exposure. Thus, a specific SMQ may be designed to support a "broad" search, useful for identifying a possible cohort of reports, or it may support a "narrow" search, useful when increased specificity is needed to identify probable reports with greater certainty than a "broad" search. The latter approach is particularly useful in searching comprehensive databases that have a large number of reports with vague or non-specific event terms, as explained below.

A "narrow" search might be sufficient by itself if it identifies a reasonable number of possible case reports to perform an adequate assessment of a possible association between the condition under review and the suspect drug in question. A "narrow" search might typically confront the user with a possible need to do multiple queries, if key terms are subsequently noted to be critical for the capture of target reports. A "broad" search, however, may also not be ideal, as this may include terms that are non-specific or otherwise not indicative of the presence or absence of the condition under review. However, a "broad" search may be necessary if the condition under review involves a syndrome that is not easily recognized by health care practitioners who are not familiar with its presentation. In this instance, individual signs or symptoms of the syndrome might be reported rather than the syndrome. Thus, the rationale for selection of terms for most Candidate SMQs is to develop the "broadest reasonable" term set. The advantage of this approach is that if certain very broad terms are not desired, they can easily be excluded from a query and this can be documented in an analysis document.

Figure 1 illustrates the concepts of "broad" and "narrow" searches, as well as variant terms that may contribute to certain searches. "Core Terms" are not always diagnostic of a particular condition, but are consistently associated with the event(s) of interest, either as a direct manifestation of the event (e.g., Torsade de pointes, or hepatic necrosis) or as an outcome of the severest form of the event (e.g., sudden death, hepatic failure). "Core Terms" are ordinarily considered for inclusion in both "Broad" and "Narrow" searches. However, most events are associated not only with particular pathognomonic manifestations that would be included as "Core Terms," but also with a number of less specific terms that may be categorized as either "Less Specific Terms" (usually associated with the event but not always essential for the diagnosis of the event) or "Very Nonspecific

Terms" (signs, symptoms or outcomes that may be associated with many conditions in addition to the condition of interest). "Specific Variants" of an overall condition may denote events only associated with either the most severe form, or a specific subcategory of a condition. For example, a specific variant of hepatic toxicity that relates only to obstructive jaundice and other types of hepatotoxicity would be defined and included in the Candidate SMQ. This subset of terms might include only some of the "Core Terms," as well as selected broad nonspecific terms. A variant of "chronic cirrhotic liver disease" might be composed of "Core Terms," including "elevated transaminases," as well as "Very Nonspecific Terms," such as "edema" and less specific terms such as "ascites." These latter two terms would ordinarily not be associated with another variant of hepatotoxicity and, thus, would be selected for inclusion in a Candidate SMQ for chronic cirrhotic liver disease (but not for a Candidate SMQ for hepatic toxicity). In some cases, a Candidate SMQ may be designed to contain two or more groupings with a requirement for presence of at least one term in each group to identify relevant cases.

Figure 1. Schematic View of MedDRA Terms Included in "Narrow" and "Broad" Searches.

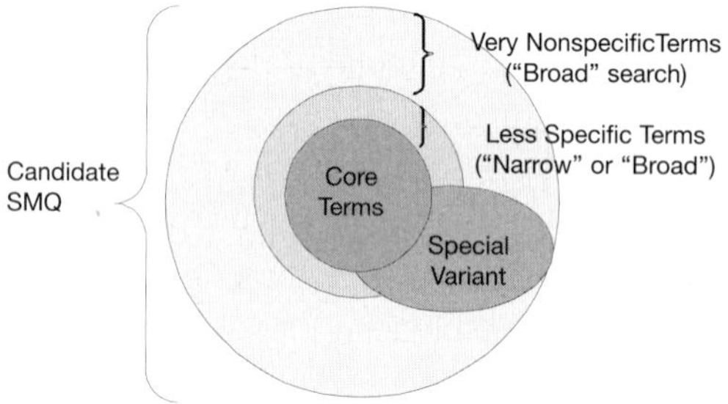

Core terms are included in both "Narrow" and "Broad" searches; Special variant terms may be included to modify a given search

8. Pre-release Testing of Candidate SMQs

Objective: Provide a level of assurance that, when applied to real data, each Candidate SMQ will identify a reasonable pool of reports to be included in a case review for the medical condition or area of interest. Since the purpose of developing SMQs is to aid in case report retrieval, the purpose of pre-release testing does not extend to any estimate of either the predictive value positive or the predictive value negative of a given SMQ. Nevertheless, successful completion of testing for each Candidate SMQ is required before that SMQ can be released to MedDRA subscribers through the ICH process.

General Approach:

1) *Phase I.* Identify eligible database(s) and identify a Responsible Tester(s) to coordinate testing. A Test Plan that includes these considerations is preferably drafted at the time assignments are made to develop new Candidate SMQs.
2) *Phase II.* The MSSO, in conjunction with the Working Group, will make Candidate SMQ specifications and associated draft documentation available to MedDRA subscribers for field-testing and comment. Any feedback received will be considered prior to formal release of each SMQ through the ICH process.

Overall responsibility for Phase I pre-release testing rests with the SMQ development team, whereas responsibility for Phase II pre-release testing is shared between the Working Group and the MSSO.

Phase I

Test articles:

Candidate SMQ: Candidate SMQ (preliminary description of MedDRA search criteria and associated draft documentation) must be agreed to by the Working Group before start of pre-release testing (NB: It may be necessary to perform some preliminary testing as part of the development of the Candidate SMQ.) Ideally, the medical literature and/or medical specialists familiar with MedDRA terminology will be consulted on an ad hoc basis to review each Candidate SMQ for clinical relevance as a retrieval tool before pre-release testing.

Marketed drug and/or biologic product(s): Since Candidate SMQs are generally intended for use in identifying problematic conditions, except for negative "controls," the medical condition or area of interest that is the target of the Candidate SMQ should be listed in the Company Core Data Sheet for each pharmaceutical product that is included in pre-release testing. When feasible, pharmaceutical products with lower rather than higher reporting rates of the target condition should be considered. For each Candidate SMQ, it is preferred that testing be conducted against more than one pharmacological category of pharmaceutical product whenever feasible. It is important to consider more than one category of product, since different drug-associated conditions may manifest themselves in slightly different ways from one group of products to another. The various types of hepatic conditions are known examples. If a pharmaceutical product can be identified that has previously been reviewed for the target condition and that review did not find a signal of an association between the pharmaceutical product and the target condition, i.e., a negative control, such product can be included in pre-release testing. Pharmaceutical products may include antibiotics, traditional medicinals, biologics (which might include monoclonal antibodies, cytokines, blood-derived products, or vaccines, etc.). The Candidate SMQ must be made available for voluntary testing in each of the ICH regions. Even though Candidate SMQs are made available, however, there is no assurance that the desired testing will be conducted in each of the ICH Regions. The Responsible Tester(s) will ensure that all products are anonymized in any data presented.

Databases: Each database selected must have adverse events coded in MedDRA (with target granularity at the Lowest Level Term or Preferred Term level). The Responsible Tester(s) will ensure that each database selected for testing is applicable for the medical condition or area of interest that is the target of the Candidate SMQ. In addition, the Responsible Tester(s) will ensure harmonization between the MedDRA version of cases in the database and the MedDRA version of the Candidate SMQ.

Test Runs: In conjunction with the SMQ development team, the Responsible Tester(s) will coordinate test runs of the Candidate SMQ, analyze results, and make recommendations to refine the Candidate SMQ based on results (expected and unexpected). The adverse events for the case reports returned must be reviewed to ensure that the intended purpose of the Candidate SMQ is met, i.e., terms should be appropriate for a "broad" search, a "narrow" search, a "broadest reasonable" search or other search subcategories as described in the supporting Candidate SMQ description. A "hit" is not required for each MedDRA term included in the Candidate SMQ for any given test product. Fine-tuning of the Candidate SMQ may require several iterations.

Results:

Design aspects of the specific pre-release testing plan and results of testing, including any adjustments to the Candidate SMQ, should be documented in a consistent and transparent format. For example, if a test run includes a term that yields a high number of irrelevant or marginally relevant cases, it may be desirable to delete that term to reduce the "noise" level.

Interpretation:

The Candidate SMQ development team must define criteria for acceptance and non-acceptance of the results of testing. The acceptance criteria, which should be defined for each SMQ, along with results of testing, will be reviewed and must be approved by the Working Group. An anonymized summary of pre-release testing should ordinarily be included in the Methodology section that describes each SMQ and should be made available for user inspection.

Phase II

Following Phase I testing, Candidate SMQs will be made available to all MedDRA subscribers for additional testing under field conditions. This "provisional release" by the MSSO for subscriber testing and comment will ordinarily be staggered in time from the release of official MedDRA versions and should only be used for purposes of providing feedback on Candidate SMQ development. Such a "provisional release" should not be used for regulatory purposes or decision-making. Feedback from such testing from the subscriber community, including relevant medical specialists, will be solicited by the MSSO; ordinarily it will be the responsibility of the Working Group to address any comments that concern medical concepts and the MSSO will be responsible for resolving user feedback on file format and distribution issues prior to release of the finalized SMQ.

Note: Once the MSSO releases an SMQ for use by the subscriber community, the SMQ will be subjected to routine maintenance (including the Change Request process), but no further requirement for testing by the Working Group or the MSSO is anticipated.

9. Modification of SMQs

It is the intention of the Working Group that SMQs should ordinarily be applied in full and without modification by users, although where optional lists of terms are built into the SMQ, the user may choose which lists to apply and then should specify the details in an analysis document. However, the selected lists should be used in their entirety. When case reports have been identified and retrieved, it may then be acceptable for users to eliminate reports that, on review of the case description, are not relevant to the specific issue in question. In these circumstances, it is expected that the user will state the number and identity of excluded reports, and detailed reasons for their exclusion.

Under certain circumstances, it may be appropriate for the user to tailor the SMQ for the purposes of the particular search required. If such customization is undertaken, it is important that the user is transparent in reporting results as the product of a non-standard search based on an SMQ (rather than describing the results as a product of an SMQ).

10. Limitations

SMQs developed by the Working Group are the result of individual and small group initiative, followed by Working Group consensus. Inevitably, there may be differences of opinion about the value of including a particular term or collection of terms. Thus, SMQs may not be comprehensive, error-free, or universally applicable. However, an important consideration is that SMQs represent a Standardised approach that should yield reproducible results.

MedDRA versions present a special challenge in the development of SMQs. The rubric attached to each SMQ identifies the particular version of MedDRA that was used by the Working Group in development activities. Subsequent versions of MedDRA, by definition, have not been used in constructing the search. However, during the process of maintaining MedDRA and the SMQs, the MSSO will update each SMQ, producing an equivalent SMQ (version) for each MedDRA version. If the database in use does not contain the same version of MedDRA stipulated for the search, results may be different from that intended by the Working Group. This is because PT level terms may be demoted to LLTs, or could be moved from one SOC location to another; new secondary linkages could be added, or different MedDRA groupings of terms could be created as part of the routine MedDRA maintenance process. Hence, a different list of terms could have been included in an SMQ produced at another time. It should be a matter of good practice for any database search to include a statement of the version of MedDRA utilized, together with a descriptive statement concerning coding conventions used and the policy for updating the database (or not) with the release of new versions of MedDRA. Note, however, that one purpose of MedDRA maintenance is to ensure that existing SMQs are updated to match the current version of MedDRA; the user should be able to select the correct version of the SMQ for the MedDRA version in the subject database. This will not remedy any differences within or across databases that result from variations in coding conventions or their application. Further, it should be noted that the Working Group specifies English as the base language to be used in developing Candidate SMQs. Thus, translation-related factors may impact the results obtained from the application of an SMQ to data from non-English language reports or to databases coded with non-English language versions of MedDRA.

III. APPLICATION OF STANDARDISED MedDRA QUERIES (SMQs) IN PHARMACOVIGILANCE

1. Introduction

When conducting search queries in a pharmacovigilance database, it is critical for all stakeholders (e.g,. companies and regulators) to be reviewing data that have been analysed in a consistent fashion. In this respect, a comprehensive list of MedDRA terms that relate to a specific adverse drug reaction (ADR) or clinical safety issue is key so that informed decisions can be taken.

The use of Standardised MedDRA Queries (SMQs) will apply to all aspects of such evaluations from pre-approval clinical trials to post-approval studies and contribute to a comprehensive evaluation of benefit and risk.

Standard statistical approaches used in pharmacovigilance which tend to utilise a specific PT could be looked into by using an SMQ instead. The methods such as Bayesian techniques or proportional reporting ratios could be applied over time in order to identify and follow-up specific signals or areas where the number of case reports received are higher than expected from background data.

This approach could already start at the time of authorisation and is in line with international initiatives (e.g. pharmacovigilance planning) such as the CIOMS VI and ICH E2E initiatives that aim at the proactive involvement of pharmacovigilance throughout the product life-cycle.

2. Clinical Trials

At the planning stage of clinical trials to be conducted pre- or post-approval when protocols are drafted a well-defined MedDRA SMQ should be used with respect to any safety area to be monitored and analysed. For instance, if the medicinal product is being investigated for hepatotoxicity, the relevant SMQ for this clinical safety issue should be stated and fully referenced in the study protocol.

Clinical trials being conducted to support the initial authorisation or thosc concentrating on efficacy, e.g., new indications, do not routinely come under the scope of SMQs. This is because safety aspects are adequately investigated by close monitoring of suspected adverse events including causality assessments and expedited reporting as appropriate. These aspects are best covered in the final study reports. There will be situations, however, for which safety issues emerging in the post-approval period will necessitate review of all safety data, i.e., clinical trial and pre- and post-approval pharmacovigilance reports. Under such circumstances, SMQs can be applied to all these data in the overall safety analysis.

3. Pharmacovigilance

The use of SMQs is applicable to all stages of the pharmacovigilance process as follows:

3.1 At authorisation

Clinical trials that are planned to support marketing authorisation as well as pre- and post-authorisation safety studies or risk management programmes may be suitable for application of SMQs used in order to analyse possible safety issues. This means that clinical study reports, summaries and expert reports generated in the post-approval period should adopt a consistent method in terms of MedDRA SMQs. When comparisons in safety profile are made between different products or at different times, the same methodology should be used in terms of SMQ so as to reach valid conclusions.

3.2 Post-marketing surveillance

Definition and consistent application of SMQs will be key towards signal detection in order to retrieve cases for further evaluation. This applies not only to spontaneous resports of adverse drug reactions but also to all types of epidemiological studies, post-authorisation studies and, when appropriate, risk management programmes put in place during the post-approval period, when these are targeted to clinical safety issues.

3.3 Benefit:risk evaluation

By extension, MedDRA SMQs will apply to the evaluation of safety and benefit:risk balance of medicinal products. Where there is a specific outcome (e.g., sudden death, liver transplant etc.) that could impact the output of relevant searches, these searches should include such outcomes. The choice of a broad or narrow search strategy will depend on the particular issue under evaluation and the choice of specificity or sensitivity needed in the analyses.

4. Profiling

Use of a consistent approach using SMQs will provide an opportunity for profiling individual medicines as regards to clinical safety.

The characteristic safety profile could be determined at the time of the marketing authorisation. Subsequently, the "evolving" profile could be developed on the basis of additional data from spontaneous reports as well as additional studies, including epidemiology.

There is potential for SMQs to screen for safety signals at different levels of the MedDRA hierarchy e.g. SOC/HLGT/HLT/PT level.

IV. The Development of Search Strategies

This section reviews general aspects of the concept of data retrieval from safety databases as far as they relate to SMQs and discusses important elements of the methods used by the CIOMS Working Group for the development of SMQs.

Safety database queries covered by SMQs

In the context of SMQs, database queries refer to searches in a drug safety database for cases of adverse events (AEs) relevant to a specified medical condition. The factors determining these searches are principally medical in nature. Other parameters, such as date of occurrence of AEs, patient's age and gender, and event outcome may be essential elements of the search, but are not covered by the concept of SMQs. Also other factors, such as disease severity, drug names and patient demographics that are not part of MedDRA are excluded from the SMQ.

Database queries using SMQs can be used for a number of purposes[1] which principally comprise the following:

- Responses to queries about specific aspects of marketed medicines or investigational compounds raised by regulatory authorities, health professionals or the manufacturer, etc.
- Comparisons of the frequency of the occurrence of specified medical conditions between individual products or groups of products including execution of a signal detection process.
- Evaluations of safety issues arising while preparing safety summaries for license applications or investigating possible safety signals for marketed products.
- Formal reviews of identified safety issues for periodic safety update reports, expert reports, the preparation of reference safety information documents, etc.

Factors affecting the quality of safety database queries using MedDRA

Because MedDRA is a complex and large terminology, the most important factors affecting the quality of search results are probably determined by the extent to which the persons performing the search understand MedDRA and by their familiarity with medical terminology and medical conditions.

Other factors affecting search results depend upon the way that the organisations have chosen to implement MedDRA including the way that legacy data have been migrated. Query results might differ for data coded ab *initio* using MedDRA, compared with data where terms previously coded using a legacy terminology were assigned MedDRA codes. Another cause for differences relates to the fact that contrary to relevant guidelines[2], some organisations select for each individual case the SOC which they consider primary depending on the context or according to drug or clinical trial project. Also the method for term selection at the time of coding and data entry may be important, for example, whether signs, symptoms, investigations and diagnosis are recorded for a particular AE or only the diagnosis.

Apart from practices determined by the organisation, the database itself may determine some aspects of search results: the version of MedDRA used, whether the safety database is updated with each new version of MedDRA, and whether data already on the database are changed in line with the new versions. The structure of the safety database, including the levels of MedDRA used and whether multiaxiality (secondary SOC linkages) are incorporated. Databases also vary in their capability to accept the MedDRA data model and automatic allocation of MedDRA locations and upward linkages from LLT within the database may not be feasible.

In addition the results of a search are critically affected by the method used in its performance. Thus, the use of multiaxiality in searching helps to increase the yield of relevant terms, but multiaxial linkages in MedDRA may not be comprehensive[3]. Hence, these cannot be relied on as a substitute for medical knowledge and understanding. Another consideration is the level of terms used in the query – is the search based upon Preferred Terms, terms from a different level or from a mixture of levels.

How are safety database queries generated?

Although a query may be based on the selection of terms used in a particular database under review, this is not a valid approach for generally applicable searches since such a search is only valid for the given database and only at the given point in time.

Generally applicable search queries are based on the entire terminology used for coding[3,4]. Only if the search parameters are independent of the database can the query be applied to any database which uses this terminology. The SMQs prepared by the CIOMS Working Group therefore utilise this approach. Because the queries are, by definition, based on MedDRA terms, their content is dependent upon the version of MedDRA used. SMQs are updated by the MSSO for each new version of MedDRA and it is necessary for the user to ascertain that the MedDRA version of the search and of the database used are consistent.

Development of SMQs by the working group

Although, as discussed in the Overview section, details of the methods used by the CIOMS Working Group in preparing each of the specific SMQs are discussed in the explanatory text for that SMQ there are some general common rules which are applied for the preparation of all SMQs.

Before starting the selection of MedDRA terms:

- Establishment of a clear definition of the safety issue(s) or the adverse reaction(s) to be investigated by the proposed SMQ by using standard medical textbooks and the CIOMS publication on Definitions of Terms and Criteria for their use[5] (if a definition is available).
- Clear definition of the scope of the search. Decision on whether the SMQ should be broad (i.e. intended to capture all possible cases, whilst possibly including some that may be irrelevant) or narrow (i.e. intended to capture only the cases most likely to represent the condition under review) or whether it should provide queries for both of these types.
- Decision whether additional less specific searches are required in certain situations e.g. a search for renal impairment in addition to a search on renal failure, or a search on myopathy in addition to a search on rhabdomyolysis. In some instances a number of interrelated searches need to be developed in order to provide for a comprehensive evaluation of terms related to broad subject e.g. hepatic toxicity.

Methods used for the compilation of terms:

- It is essential that a flexible approach is used and that medical common sense prevails over a purely mechanistic method.
- Inclusion and exclusion criteria need to be clearly specified. Normal and unspecified investigation terms should be excluded.
- For the search for terms in the dictionary a dual method is usually applied consisting of a bottom-up and a top-down approach. Both

should be applied at some point in the process in order not to miss relevant terms. For the bottom-up approach a series of searches across all SOCs is performed for MedDRA LLTs that are relevant to the query. This is followed by identification of the PTs to which these terms link and their super-ordinate group terms (HLTs, HLGTs and SOCs). A focused top-down exploration of the MedDRA tree is carried out looking for additional relevant PTs under the group terms that were initially identified.

- During the initial stage of the search definition, both primary and secondary locations of relevant PTs are scrutinized in the multi-axial approach. However when presenting the data in the final SMQ only primary locations are listed.
- During the preparation of a new SMQ the MedDRA version used by all contributors must be the same and clearly stated.
- Three MedDRA SOCs need to be screened routinely for any new SMQ: Investigations, Surgical and medical procedures, and General disorders and administration site conditions.
- Algorithms are not usually necessary for SMQs apart from situations where a syndrome of clinical findings is likely to involve a collection of PTs, some of which are common to many other medical conditions, hence non-specific (e.g. the cardinal symptoms of anaphylaxis). In such situations additional searches using combinations of PTs may be warranted in order to improve specificity (and prevent the retrieval of excessive numbers of reports from a database that may not be relevant). Some SMQs therefore provide options for the use of combinations of terms if the inclusion of a term on its own may be too non-specific, whereas its use in combination with one or more additional terms is more likely to identify relevant reports.

Additional comments:

- If, as ordinarily required, the proposed SMQ was tested using a pharmacovigilance database during its development this should be clearly described including methodology and relevant results.
- If during the initial screening for relevant PTs it is realised that some LLTs but not their corresponding PT may be relevant for the SMQ, thus indicating that the given LLT and its PT represent different medical concepts, the MSSO should be informed to consider upgrading these specific LLTs to PTs.

Sensitivity and specificity of searches

It is necessary to refer to the characteristics of each search in respect of its degree of sensitivity and specificity. The greater the sensitivity (or breadth), the higher is the likelihood of finding all cases of the medical condition in question. Increasing the sensitivity of a search can be done by adding terms for signs, symptoms and investigational findings that may represent the medical condition even in the absence of a diagnosis. Such an approach may, however, lead to the retrieval of other conditions with different aetiologies thus decreasing specificity. For example, a search for cases of ventricular tachyarrhythmia might include the term seizure. However, although seizures can be caused by ventricular tachyarrhythmia and may be the sole clinical presentation such a search will also retrieve reports of seizures due to other, non-cardiac causes. Broad, highly sensitive searches therefore increase the likelihood of identifying all cases of the condition in question, but also the likelihood of retrieving irrelevant cases[6]. A balance needs to be found between completeness and discriminatory value. If common symptoms with many causes, such as nausea or dizziness, are included in a query, the noise will probably be detrimental to the search.

The specificity of a search, on the other hand, indicates the likelihood that it will identify only cases that contain the medical condition under review. A highly specific search may focus on a small number of terms in MedDRA that represent the precise condition. It will, however, not identify relevant cases reporting terms for the relevant signs, symptoms and investigations only without the diagnosis. If, for example, a search for cases of complete heart block excludes the PT Atrioventricular block and the PT Conduction disorder, relevant cases that were incompletely reported might not be identified.

Many SMQs provide options for broad and for narrow searches.

Customising searches

If search results are reported referring to a SMQ, these should be applied in full and without modification by the users. Some SMQs provide specific sub-searches which if selected should also be clearly specified by the user and the selected sub-searches should be used in their entirety. However, after cases have been identified and retrieved by the SMQ, it may be acceptable to eliminate those that, on review are found not to be relevant to the specific issue in question. It is, however, expected that details of this procedure are described in the report.

If, under certain circumstances, it is necessary for the user to tailor an SMQ for the purposes of a particular question, it is not acceptable to refer to the results of this search as relating to a given SMQ.

Limitations

The searches performed by the Working Group are the result of individual initiative, followed by group consensus. Inevitably, there may be differences of opinion about the value of including a particular term or collection of terms. However, one of the key benefits of using these queries is the fact that they are "standardised". That is not to say that they are comprehensive, error-free or universally acceptable, only that performing one of these searches on a database should be reproducible and that an identical search may be performed on any database utilising the appropriate version of MedDRA.

References

1. Brown EG and Douglas S (2000). Tabulation and analysis of pharmacovigilance data using the Medical Dictionary for Regulatory Activities. Pharmacoepidemiology and Drug Safety 9, 479-489.
2. MedDRA Term Selection: Points to Consider. ICH-Endorsed Guide for MedDRA Users.
3. Brown EG (2003). Methods and pitfalls in searching drug safety databases utilising the Medical Dictionary for Regulatory Activities (MedDRA) Drug Safety 26(3): 145-158.
4. Fescharek R, Dechert G, Reichert D, et al (1996). Overall analysis of spontaneously reported adverse events: a worthwhile exercise or flogging a dead horse? Pharmaceutical Medicine 10: 71-86.
5. Reporting Adverse Drug Reactions – Definitions of Terms and Criteria for their use. CIOMS, Geneva 1999.
6. Goldman SA (2002). Adverse event reporting and standardizing medical terminologies: strengths and limitations. Drug Inf J 36: 439-444.

V. Template Concerning Communication of Search Results

The CIOMS Working Group on Standardised MedDRA Queries has proposed guidelines for identifying safety case reports that may be relevant to specific medical conditions. One approach to case selection involves use of Standardised queries that have been defined by the CIOMS Working Group. Alternatively, the search strategy may involve creation of a database query or set of queries constructed *de novo* from terms in the MedDRA hierarchy. The following points should be considered when communicating the search strategy selected and the results obtained using either Standardised or customized searches.

This includes a description of the methodology used for the selection of the data in such a way that the process is clear, transparent, and can be accurately and easily reproduced by someone else or at a future time (i.e., retraceable and able to withstand the scrutiny of an audit). In addition to a description of how the information obtained from the database search was analyzed, information on the reason for conducting the search should also be included. It is also important to include background information on the drug and the adverse event(s) of interest.

Below is an outline of points that might be included when communicating results of pharmacovigilance database searches.

Communication of Search Results

1. Executive Summary

This section should be a very brief summary that includes the name of the subject drug, a statement of the question and its source, an overview of the search strategy and database; summary results from the search, and an overall conclusion.

2. Background Information

2.1 Introduction

This section should cover the following topics: Request source, specific request, history of request, current position of company (in company label or not), objectives of current report.

2.2 Background on the Drug

In case it is a "stand alone document", relevant information on the drug should be included here on indication, formulation, dose and schedule, mechanism of action, other background on drug, etc. (e.g. taken from the package insert).

In some instances it may be desirable to present other information in this section, such as population exposure estimates, to put the number of reported events into perspective.

2.3 Background on Medical Condition, Adverse Event, or Group of Disorders

The adverse event / group of disorders (e.g. Stevens-Johnson syndrome / cardiac disorders) being assessed must be clearly defined. This can be an overview as would be presented in a textbook or review paper. The information should be referenced.

3. Methodology

3.1 Data extraction

3.1.1 Source of Information

The source of information (e.g., the specific safety database or databases) should be described, preferably using a standard text. The types of case reports reviewed should be specified, e.g., spontaneous, clinical trial, related, unrelated, serious, non-serious, medically confirmed, non-medically confirmed, etc, as may be relevant. In case of in-licensed products, companies involved, information on responsibility for the database (one or several companies), source(s) of information entered onto the database(s) should be included.

3.1.2. Search and Selection Strategy

The precise scope of the search is defined here. The version of MedDRA (installed on the database) being used for the search must be specified. If a Standardised MedDRA Query (SMQ) is used, the name and version (including MedDRA version it is based upon) should also be indicated. In case of a modification of a SMQ, a rationale for inclusion/exclusion criteria concerning certain event terms should be given to justify the resulting data set.

It is recommended that a full list of case identifiers of all retrieved cases should be provided in the text or as an appendix. The reason for this is that we are dealing with live databases. This will allow to identify cases that have been deleted later on (e.g. because it was identified to be a duplicate of another case), or underwent a change in adverse event term.

In case a previous analysis has been done for the same drug and not exactly the same search strategy is being used (e.g., a SMQ is being used for the first time; another terminology was used due to the switch from WHOART to MedDRA; an updated MedDRA version is used; change in coding conventions; or a wider approach), describe here the changes in the search strategy compared to the previous retrieval.

3.2 Medical Analysis

This section should describe how the extracted data were analyzed and should include the definition of the criteria used for the medical evaluation of the cases chosen from the data extracted above. The method for classification / stratification of results should be provided.

4. Results

4.1 Information from Safety Database

4.1.1 Overview

This section should include an overview and summary of the data, including the cut-off date for the search. Graphical displays (flow chart or graph) can be of benefit, especially if the number of cases retrieved is large, to provide the reader with a quick overview of the results. Summary tables can then supply demographic data. The overview may include total number of similar cases / number of similar events, serious cases and deaths as well as a summary of relevant information regarding demographics, sources, countries of report versus sales, number of cases per year, relevant sub-groups, etc.

4.1.2 Case Presentation

Depending on the number of cases retrieved, narratives, tables, or a combination of both might be appropriate for presentation in this section.

4.1.3 Summary of Data

In case a large number of cases was reviewed, it might be appropriate to provide a summary of results highlighting relevant information. This is intended to provide a summary of the case series that has been identified from the search of the database, with an evaluation of the strength of the cases and the company assessment of those data.

4.2 Additional relevant information

There may be additional information that the author of the report may wish to disclose, such as late-breaking information, results of clinical trials, information from scientific literature, epidemiological studies, findings from preclinical studies, background rates of the medical condition under study or information on reference products.

5. Discussion and Conclusion

Details of the results of data searches are presented in the result section. This section should be reserved for interpretation of the results and an overall conclusion. Evidence from literature can be included here to support interpretation; information already provided in the background section can be cross-referenced.

The impact of the analysis on the overall medical assessment of the product safety profile may be summarized here and may include recommendations for additional work or other specific actions.

VI. Examples of Candidate SMQs

Torsade de Pointes/QT Prolongation

**This SMQ is not for routine use.
It is only an example.**

Introduction

This Standardised MedDRA Query (SMQ) was developed as part of the joint effort between the CIOMS Working Party on Standardised MedDRA Queries and the MedDRA MSSO to develop standard sets of MedDRA terms to identify possible cases of several problematic, often drug-related adverse events that are sometimes observed during post-marketing experience. This specific query is intended to identify relevant MedDRA terms to search for cases of possible *torsade de pointes* or QT prolongation.

Background on *Torsade de Pointes*

Torsade de pointes (TdP) is a form of rapid ventricular tachycardia.[1-6] The underlying cause of *torsade de pointes* appears to be related to delayed ventricular repolarization, primarily resulting from blockade of potassium conductance.[2,5] This can be hereditary (eg congenital long QT syndrome), in which case it involves genetic abnormalities of cardiac potassium or sodium channels involved in repolarization. It can also be acquired, in which case it may be caused by electrolyte disturbances (particularly hypokalemia and hypomagnesemia), intracranial events (such as sub-arachnoid hemorrhage), myocarditis, hypothyroidism, arsenic poisoning, liquid protein diets, bradyarrhythmias (particularly third-degree AV block), and a variety of drugs that appear to block potassium conductance channels (such as type Ia and III antiarrhythmics, phenothiazines, tricyclic antidepressants, macrolide antibiotics, and some of the non-sedating H_1-selective antihistamines).[1-6] Furthermore, in some cases of acquired torsade de pointes, there appears to be a genetic predisposition related to sub-clinical potassium channel abnormalities that can become unmasked following the precipitating event or exposure.[2,5]

On electrocardiogram (ECG), *torsade de pointes* is characterized by polymorphic QRS complexes that change in amplitude and cycle length.[1-6] Other ECG changes that are associated with or precede onset of *torsade de pointes* include prolonged QT or QTc interval (usually >500-600msec or >440msec respectively in patients experiencing *torsade de pointes*), prominent U waves, T wave alternans or bizarre T wave aberrations, or "long-short sequences" (characterized by a long QT interval ending in a ventricular ectopic beat followed by a short sequence ending in a sinus beat with marked TU changes).[1-6] The arrhythmia can resolve spontaneously, but acquired forms often recur until the underlying cause is corrected, and can progress to ventricular fibrillation.[1-4] Clinical manifestations during prolonged episodes can include episodes of palpitations, dizziness, syncope, and, rarely, sudden death; however, patients are often unaware of palpitations.[1,2,5,6]

Methodology

The MedDRA terms used were identified as a result of a "bottom up" search via Lowest Level Terms (LLTs) to identify what specific MedDRA (version 5.1) Preferred Terms (PTs) would be encoded for cases reporting events possibly associated with this syndrome, and what System Organ Classes (SOCs) these PTs are listed under. In order to make this search reasonably sensitive, the reported events for which MedDRA PTs were searched for included *torsade de pointes*, QT/QTc prolongation, ventricular arrhythmia/fibrillation/flutter/ tachycardia, U- or T-wave abnormalities, syncope, and sudden death. After the relevant MedDRA PTs and their place in the MedDRA hierarchy were identified, a "top down" review was performed to identify other related, potentially relevant PTs, as well as their primary pathways.

In an effort to determine how well the proposed MedDRA search query would identify potential cases of *torsade de pointes* and/or QT prolongation, Pfizer's early alert safety database was searched using the proposed search strategy. Pfizer's early alert safety database contains cases of adverse events reported spontaneously to Pfizer, cases reported from health authorities, cases published in the medical literature, and cases of serious adverse events reported from clinical studies and Pfizer-sponsored marketing programs (solicited cases) regardless of causality. The database was reviewed for non-clinical study origin cases reported by health care professionals to the database through 31 March 2003 for five Pfizer products. *Torsade de pointes* and/or QT prolongation were documented for two of these products at the time that they were commercially introduced (hereafter referred to as Compound 1 and Compound 2), and, as a result, have been the subject of vigorous post-marketing surveillance. *Torsade de pointes* and/or QT prolongation were recently added to the core data sheet for the third product (hereafter referred to as Compound 3) based on cases reported during this product's post-marketing experience. For the fourth product (hereafter referred to as Compound 4), *torsade de pointes* and/or QT prolongation have been reported in association with pharmacokinetic drug interactions with drugs such as cisapride, but has not generally been thought to be associated with these events by itself; however, there have been a few published case reports of *torsade de pointes* and/or QT prolongation that the reporters thought not to be the result of drug interactions. The fifth product (hereafter referred to as Compound 5) is not currently thought to be associated with these events; however, another member of the same pharmacologic class has recently been identified as possibly being associated with QT prolongation. A subsequent recent re-evaluation of this issue for Compound 5 confirmed that it does not appear to be associated with *torsade de pointes* and/or QT prolongation. For these products, it was expected that the proposed search strategy would identify a reasonable pool of potential cases to be included in a case review.

Results and Discussion

As a result of this review of the MedDRA dictionary (version 5.1), a total of 22 relevant PTs were identified. The primary pathway for these 22 PTs has them listed under five SOCs, five High Level Group Terms (HLGTs), and six High Level Terms (HLTs). These terms are listed in Table 1.

In an effort to make this standard query relatively specific, not all possibly *torsade de pointes*- or QT prolongation-related events were included. For example, PTs for events such as palpitations, dizziness, or events suggestive of non-specific ECG changes were not included. These events are often non-serious, too non-specific, and are often reported as the only potentially related events in many cases. In such cases where these are the only potentially relevant event terms, review of these case can be expected to be uninformative as they are unlikely to contain sufficient information to contribute meaningful information.

Based on the PTs identified, queries of the database to identify relevant cases for review were conducted in a two-step manner. The first step was to conduct a "narrow" search to identify a "core" set of cases specifically reported to involve *torsade de pointes* or QT prolongation, and would include the PTs Long QT syndrome, Long QT syndrome congenital, *Torsade de pointes*, Ventricular tachycardia (because of the LLTs TdP ventricular tachycardia and Polymorphic ventricular tachycardia), Electrocardiogram QT corrected interval prolonged, and Electrocardio-gram QT prolonged. The second step was to conduct a broad search to identify cases reporting PTs that might involve cardiac-related events often associated with *torsade de pointes* or QT prolongation or, since syncope is often the presenting symptom, possible syncope-related neurologic sequelae of *torsade de pointes*. The broader search would include the PTs Cardiac arrest, Cardiac fibrillation NOS, Cardio-respiratory arrest, Ventricular arrhythmia NOS, Ventricular fibrillation, Ventricular flutter, Electrocardiogram U-wave abnormality, Electrocardiogram U-wave biphasic, Electrocardiogram repolarisation abnormality, Cardiac death, Sudden cardiac death, and Sudden death, Loss of consciousness, Syncope, Syncope aggravated, and Vasovagal attack.

The results of the searches of Pfizer's early alert safety database for the five test products are summarized in Tables 2, 3, and 4. A listing of the number of cases reporting each of the relevant MedDRA PTs is presented in Table 2. The number of cases identified by the narrow search and the number of cases added after the broad search is presented in Table 3.

In Table 4, the cases identified are further characterized by the presence of other PTs reported in the same case. The cases identified by the narrow search are categorized as to whether the narrow search PTs were the only relevant reported PTs or if they also reported broad search PTs. The cases reporting broad PTs that did not report narrow PTs are categorized as to whether the broad PT was also reported with PTs suggestive of other events that might be associated with *torsade de pointes* or QT prolongation (such as hypokalemia, myocarditis, bradyarrhythmias, intracranial events, or thyroid disorders) and could involve *torsade de pointes* or QT prolongation. The cases reporting broad PTs without narrow PTs were also categorized as to whether they were reported together with relevant, but non-*torsade de pointes* or non-QT prolongation-related events (such as seizures, myocardial infarction or other events suggestive of myocardial ischemia, pulmonary embolism, non-QT-related arrhythmias, hypoglycemia, and hypotension and/or orthostasis), or if the reported broad PTs were the only reported events or only relevant reported events. In the latter instance, it is unlikely that the cases contain sufficient information to determine if the reported broad PTs were possibly the result of *torsade de pointes* or QT prolongation.

For the two products known to be associated with *torsade de pointes* and/or QT prolongation when they were commercially introduced (Compounds 1 and 2), most of the cases (250 of 278 and 129 of 172 respectively) were identified by the narrow search. Very few cases (2 and 4 respectively) reporting broad search PTs also reported PTs for other events associated with *torsade de pointes* or QT prolongation, and very few (8 and 20 respectively) reported broad search PTs that might have been related to other non-*torsade de pointes* and/or non-QT prolongation-related events; the broad search PTs were the only relevant reported events in 18 and 19 cases respectively. Thus, for drug products clearly associated with *torsade de pointes* and/or QT prolongation, the proposed SMQ adequately identified cases of *torsade de pointes* and/or QT prolongation.

For Compound 3, for which *torsade de pointes* and/or QT prolongation was recently added to the core data sheet based on cases reporting during its post-marketing experience, about one-third of all cases identified by the proposed SMQ (70 of 219) were identified by the narrow search. An additional 17 cases involved broad search PTs with other events possibly related to *torsade de pointes* and/or QT prolongation. The remaining cases were approximately equally distributed between those for which broad search PTs were the only relevant reported events (69 cases) or where the reported broad search PTs were possibly associated with non-*torsade de pointes* and/or non-QT prolongation-related events (63 cases). For Compound 4, which may be associated with *torsade de pointes* and/or QT prolongation related to drug interactions but not by itself, about half of all cases identified by the proposed SMQ (90 of 189) were found by the narrow search. An additional 18 cases reported broad search PTs with other events associated with *torsade de pointes* and/or QT prolongation. Similar, smaller numbers of cases were identified that reported broad search PTs as either the only relevant reported event (38 cases) or where the reported broad search PTs could have been associated with other, non-*torsade de pointes* and/or non-QT prolongation-related events (43 cases). These results suggest that the SMQ should be reasonably efficient at identifying relevant cases of *torsade de pointes* and/or QT prolongation for products that were not thought to be associated with these events when first commercially introduced, but were subsequently found to be associated with *torsade de pointes* and/or QT prolongation during those products' post-marketing experience.

For Compound 5, which is not thought to be associated with *torsade de pointes* and/or QT prolongation, 30 cases were identified by the narrow search compared to a total of 500 cases identified by both the narrow and broad searches; however, of the cases identified by the narrow search the only reported narrow search PT was Ventricular tachycardia, and none of these 30 cases encoded to the LLTs TdP ventricular tachycardia or Polymorphic ventricular tachycardia. A similar number of cases (34) reporting broad search PTs also reported PTs for other events associated with *torsade de pointes* or QT prolongation. In total then, 64 cases reported either narrow search PTs or broad search PTs with other events suggestive of *torsade de pointes* and/or QT prolongation. The vast majority of cases identified by the proposed SMQ that reported broad search PTs with no narrow search PTs (436 of 470 cases) reported either the broad search PTs as the only relevant reported events (233 cases), in which case it is unlikely that the cases contain sufficient information to determine if the reported broad PTs were possibly the result of *torsade de pointes* or QT prolongation, or also reported other events (203 cases) for which the reported broad search PTs might have been related. This is not entirely unexpected for Compound 5, as it is indicated for use in a patient population that has multiple cardiovascular risk factors possibly associated with the occurrence of events that would map to many of the broad search PTs, and is associated with hypotension and related events that might have syncope-related events as sequelae. While the total number of cases suggestive of *torsade de pointes* and/or QT prolongation based only on the nature of the reported PTs was small (64) for Compound 5, it represents a reasonably sized pool of cases for review to determine if there is a signal of risk for *torsade de pointes* and/or QT prolongation being associated with this product.

Summary and Conclusions

The MedDRA dictionary (version 5.1) was reviewed to identify search terms for inclusion in an SMQ to identify cases of potential *torsade de pointes* and/or QT prolongation. This review identified a total of 22 relevant PTs. The primary pathway for these 22 PTs has them listed under four SOCs, four high level group terms (HLGTs), and five high level terms (HLTs). These 22 PTs can be divided into terms for inclusion in a narrow search to identify cases specifically reported to involve *torsade de pointes* and/or QT prolongation, and a broad search to identify cases reporting PTs that might involve cardiac-related events often associated with *torsade de pointes* or QT prolongation or, since syncope is often the presenting symptom, possible syncope-related neurologic sequelae of *torsade de pointes*.

The SMQ was tested against five products, two of which were documented to be associated with *torsade de pointes* and/or QT prolongation when they were commercially introduced, one of which had recently had *torsade de pointes* and/or QT prolongation added to its core data sheet based on cases reported during its post-marketing experience, one of which has been reported to be associated with *torsade de pointes* and/or QT prolongation as a result of a pharmacokinetic drug interaction with compounds such as cisapride, and one of which was recently reviewed to determine if it had an association with *torsade de pointes* and/or QT prolongation. The results of these tests indicate that the proposed SMQ satisfactorily identified an adequate pool of cases to be reviewed to determine if an association exists with *torsade de pointes* and/or QT prolongation for each of the five test products. Based on these results, the proposed SMQ should be satisfactory for use to identify potential non-clinical study origin cases of *torsade de pointes* and/or QT prolongation reported during any drug product's post-marketing experience.

References

1 Zipes DP. Specific arrhythmias: diagnosis and treatment. *Heart Disease: A Textbook of Cardiovascular Medicine (5th Ed).* Braunwald E (Ed). WB Sauanders: Philadelphia, 1997, pg. 640-704.

2 Marriott HJL and Conover MB. Polymorphic ventricular tachycardia. *Advanced Concepts in Arrhythmias (3rd Ed).* Mosby: New York, 1998, pg. 293-310.

3 Definitions and basic requirements for the use of terms for reporting adverse drug reactions (XI): cardiovascular system disorders. *Pharmacoepidemiology and Drug Safety* 1998; 7:351-357.

4 Torsade de pointes. *Reporting Adverse Drug Reactions: Definitions of Terms and Criteria for Their Use.* Bankowski Z, Bruppacher R, Crusius I et al (Eds). Council for International Organizations of Medical Sciences: Geneva, 1999, pg. 81-82.

5 Josephson ME and Zimetbaum P. The tachyarrhythmias. *Harrison's Principles of Internal Medicine (15th Ed).* Braunwald E, Fauci AS, Kasper DL et al (Eds). McGraw-Hill: New York, 2001, pg. 1292-1309.

6 Bauman JL and Schoen MD. Arrhythmias. *Pharmacotherapy: A Pathophysiologic Approach (5th Ed).* DiPiro JT, Talbert RL, Yee GC et al (Eds). McGraw-Hill: New York, 2002, pg. 273-303.

Table 1. MedDRA (version 5.1) Preferred Terms to Include for *Torsade de Pointes*/QT Prolongation (Primary Pathway Sorted by SOC, HLGT, and HLT).

System Organ Class (SOC)	High Level Group Term (HLGT)	High Level Term (HLT)	Preferred Term (PT)
Cardiac disorders	Cardiac arrhythmias	Cardiac conduction disorders	Long QT syndrome*
		Ventricular arrhythmias and cardiac arrest	Cardiac arrest†
			Cardiac fibrillation NOS†
			Cardio-respiratory arrest†
			Torsade de pointes*
			Ventricular arrhythmia NOS†
			Ventricular fibrillation†
			Ventricular flutter†
			Ventricular tachycardia*
Congenital, familial and genetic disorders	Cardiac and vascular disorders congenital	Cardiac disorders congenital NEC	Long QT syndrome congenital*
Investigations	Cardiac and vascular investigations (excl enzyme tests)	ECG investigations	Electrocardiogram QT corrected interval prolonged*
			Electrocardiogram QT prolonged*
			Electrocardiogram U-wave abnormality†
			Electrocardiogram U-wave biphasic†

(continued)

System Organ Class (SOC)	High Level Group Term (HLGT)	High Level Term (HLT)	Preferred Term (PT)
			Electrocardiogram repolarization abnormality†
General disorders and administration site conditions	Fatal outcomes	Death and sudden death	Cardiac death†
			Sudden cardiac death†
			Sudden death†
Nervous systems disorders	Neurologic disorders NEC	Disturbances in consciousness NEC	Loss of consciousness‡
			Syncope‡
			Syncope aggravated‡
			Vasovagal attack‡

* narrow search terms for event terms to identify “core” cases

† broad search terms for cardiac events often associated with *torsade de pointes* or QT prolongation

‡ broad search terms for possible syncope-related neurologic sequelae of *torsade de pointes*

Table 2. Health Care Professional, Non-Clinical Study Cases Reporting *Torsade de Pointes*/QT Prolongation – Related MedDRA Preferred Terms for Five Test Products Reported to Pfizer's Early Alert Safety Database Through 31 March 2003.

	Number of Cases				
MedDRA Preferred Term	**Compound 1**	**Compound 2**	**Compound 3**	**Compound 4**	**Compound 5**
Long QT syndrome*	—	—	—	—	—
Long QT syndrome congenital*	—	—	—	—	—
Torsade de pointes*	42	3	19	46	—
Electrocardiogram QT corrected interval prolonged*	79	73	—	3	—
Electrocardiogram QT prolonged*	94	51	33	41	—
Ventricular tachycardia*	60	6	27	36	30
Cardiac arrest†	12	8	41	56	159
Cardiac fibrillation NOS†	—	—	—	1	2
Cardio-respiratory arrest†	2	1	6	13	21
Ventricular arrhythmia NOS†	4	1	5	10	6
Ventricular fibrillation†	14	2	11	20	55
Ventricular flutter†	1	—	1	1	1
Electrocardiogram U-wave abnormality†	—	—	—	—	—
Electrocardiogram U-wave biphasic†	—	—	—	—	—

(continued)

	Number of Cases				
MedDRA Preferred Term	**Compound 1**	**Compound 2**	**Compound 3**	**Compound 4**	**Compound 5**
Electrocardiogram repolarization abnormality	—	1	—	—	—
Cardiac death†	2	—	—	—	2
Sudden cardiac death†	1	1	2	—	18
Sudden death†	3	1	5	1	28
Loss of consciousness‡	2	20	50	27	114
Syncope‡	10	19	58	21	136
Syncope aggravated‡	—	—	—	—	—
Vasovagal attack‡	2	1	6	1	10
Total Cases Meeting Any Search Criteria	**278**	**172**	**219**	**189**	**500**
Total Health Care Professional Non-Clinical Study Cases	**1,223**	**2,638**	**14,682**	**7,402**	**11,968**

* event terms for inclusion in a specific "core" search

† broad search terms for cardiac events often associated with *torsade de pointes* or QT prolongation

‡ broad search terms for possible syncope-related neurologic sequelae of *torsade de pointes*

Table 3. Number of Non-Clinical Study Cases Reported by Health Care Professionals Identified by Narrow and Broad Search for *Torsade de Pointes*/QT Prolongation-Related Events.

	Number of Cases Returned After Each Search				
Search Type	**Compound 1**	**Compound 2**	**Compound 3**	**Compound 4**	**Compound 5**
Narrow Search	250	129	70	90	30
Broad Search*	28	43	149	99	470
Total Cases Meeting Any SMQ Search Criteria	**278**	**172**	**219**	**189**	**500**
Total Health Care Professional Non-Clinical Study Cases	**1,223**	**2,638**	**14,682**	**7,402**	**11,968**

* cases reporting only broad search terms without reporting any narrow search terms

Table 4. Number of Non-Clinical Study Cases Reported by Health Care Professionals Identified by Narrow and Broad Search for *Torsade de Pointes*/QT Prolongation-Related Events Further Categorized by the Presence of Other Preferred Terms Reported in the Same Case.

	Number of Cases				
Narrow and Broad Search PTs Categorized by Presence of Other Reported PTs	**Compound 1**	**Compound 2**	**Compound 3**	**Compound 4**	**Compound 5**
Narrow PTs only	230	121	48	56	15
Narrow PTs with at least one broad cardiac and/or syncope-related PT	20	8	22	34	15
Total Cases With Narrow PTs	**250**	**129**	**70**	**90**	**30**
Broad cardiac PTs with other PTs associated with TdP/QT prolongation	2	1	7	13	16
Broad syncope-related PTs and other PTs associated with TdP/QT prolongation	—	3	9	5	16
Broad cardiac and syncope-related PTs and other PTs associated with TdP/QT prolongation	—	—	1	—	2
Total Cases With Broad PTs And Other PTs Associated With TdP/QT Prolongation	**2**	**4**	**17**	**18**	**34**
Total Cases With Search PTs Suggestive of TdP/QT Prolongation	**252**	**133**	**87**	**108**	**64**
Broad cardiac PTs only relevant reported events	16	4	19	26	105

(Continued)

Narrow and Broad Search PTs Categorized by Presence of Other Reported PTs	Number of Cases				
	Compound 1	Compound 2	Compound 3	Compound 4	Compound 5
Broad syncope-related PTs only relevant reported events	2	15	50	12	123
Broad cardiac and syncope-related PTs only relevant reported events	—	—	—	—	5
Total Cases With Broad PTs Only Relevant Reported Events	**18**	**19**	**69**	**38**	**233**
Broad cardiac PTs possibly related to other reported events	1	4	23	27	97
Broad syncope-related PTs possible related to other reported events	7	16	40	15	94
Broad cardiac and syncope-related PTs possible related to other reported events	—	—	—	1	12
Total Cases with Broad PTs Possibly Related to Other Reported Events	**8**	**20**	**63**	**43**	**203**
Total Cases Meeting SMQ Search Criteria	**278**	**172**	**219**	**189**	**500**

VI. Examples of Candidate SMQs

Rhabdomyolysis/Myopathy

**This SMQ is not for routine use.
It is only an example.**

Introduction

This Standardised MedDRA Query (SMQ) was developed as part of the joint effort between the CIOMS Working Party on Standardised MedDRA Queries and the MedDRA MSSO to develop standard sets of MedDRA terms to identify possible cases of several problematic, often drug-related adverse events that are sometimes observed during post-marketing experience. This specific query is intended to identify relevant MedDRA terms to search for cases of possible rhabdomyolysis or myopathy.

Background on Rhabdomyolysis and Myopathy

Myopathy is a disorder of striated muscle, with or without changes in muscle mass, and may be accompanied by muscle pain or tenderness.[1,2] Rhabdomyolysis is a syndrome resulting from extensive necrosis of skeletal muscle. This necrosis releases muscle contents, particularly creatine kinase (CK) and other muscle enzymes (such as aminotransferases and lactic dehydrogenase), creatinine, potassium, uric acid, myoglobin, calcium, and phosphorus into the systemic circulation.[3,4] Some cases are related to hereditary metabolic or structural abnormalities effecting skeletal muscle cells, such as disorders of glycogen and lipid metabolism.[3] However, the majority of cases occur in healthy individuals as a result of a variety of non-hereditary causes. These non-hereditary causes include such things as trauma (due to crushing injuries or excessive exercise), bacterial and/or viral infections (such as *Staphylococcus* or influenza), medications (such as HMG-CoA reductase inhibitors and antipsychotics) recreational drugs (such as cocaine, amphetamines, and alcohol), toxins (such as tetanus and some snake venoms), and ischemia.[3,5]

Clinical features of rhabdomyolysis can vary greatly. Mild forms may be self-limiting and the patients recover without noticeable sequelae. Severe forms can result in potentially life-threatening complications.[3-5] Muscle signs and symptoms usually include muscle pain, weakness, tenderness, and contractures, usually involving large muscles such as those of the calves, thighs, and lower back, but can also involve the chest, abdomen, palate and throat, and masticatory muscles. Other non-specific symptoms can include weight gain, fatigue, malaise, fever, nausea, tachycardia, and dark red or cola-coloured urine. Other, potentially serious systemic symptoms can include acute renal failure, compartment syndrome, disseminated intravascular coagulation, cardiomyopathy, and respiratory failure.[3,4]

Laboratory abnormalities usually considered indicative of rhabdomyolysis include elevated creatine kinase (CK, particularly CK-MM, considered abnormal if ≥ 10 times upper limit normal, but often ≥ 100 times upper limit normal in rhabdomyolysis), myoglobinuria (often with urine concentrations > 1g/L), and increased serum myoglobin (often up to 20 times upper normal limit). Other laboratory findings may include elevated concentrations of serum creatinine, lactic dehydrogenase, and aminotransferases. Hypocalcaemia may occur during the initial phases of rhabdomyolysis as a result of calcium deposition in necrotic muscle tissue secondary to release of large amounts of phosphorus. Potentially life-threatening hyperkalemia may occur in patients with acute renal failure. Diagnosis can be confirmed by muscle biopsy.[3-5]

Methodology

The MedDRA terms used were identified as a result of a "bottom up" search via Lowest Level Terms (LLTs) to identify what specific MedDRA (version 5.1) Preferred Terms (PTs) would be encoded for cases reporting events possibly associated with this syndrome, and what System Organ Classes (SOCs) these PTs are listed under. In order to make this search reasonably specific, the reported events for which MedDRA PTs were searched for included rhabdomyolysis or myopathy and manifestations strongly suggestive of myopathy such as myoglobinemia or myoglobinuria. After the relevant MedDRA PTs and their place in the MedDRA hierarchy were identified, a "top down" review was performed to identify other related, potentially relevant PTs, as well as their primary pathways.

Because of the wide variety of clinical manifestations associated with rhabdomyolysis or myopathy, it is possible that cases might also be reported that were not recognized as rhabdomyolysis at the time they were reported, and were reported to have involved compartment syndrome or some non-myopathy-related muscle events (such as myalgia, muscle fatigue or weakness, musculoskeletal pain or discomfort, or abnormal muscle biopsy) or other non-musculoskeletal events suggestive of possible rhabdomyolysis or myopathy (such as renal failure and related events, increased CK or other muscle enzymes, hypocalcaemia, or chromaturia). Any search criteria used needs to be reasonably sensitive enough to identify such cases, and a similar "bottom up" followed by a "top down" search was performed to identify potentially relevant PTs for cases involving such rhabdomyolysis-related events.

In an effort to determine how well the proposed MedDRA search query would identify potential cases of rhabdomyolysis or myopathy, Pfizer's early alert safety database was searched using the proposed search strategy. Pfizer's early alert safety database contains cases of adverse events reported spontaneously to Pfizer, cases reported from health authorities, cases published in the medical literature, and cases of serious adverse events reported from clinical studies and Pfizer-sponsored marketing programs (solicited cases) regardless of causality. The database was reviewed for non-clinical study origin cases reported by health care professionals to the database for two Pfizer products. Rhabdomyolysis was added to the labelling for the first product (hereafter referred to as Compound 1) after it had been commercially available for about two years. The database was reviewed for cases reporting events mapping to any of the PTs listed in the proposed SMQ through the month that the labelling was amended to include rhabdomyolysis.

For the second product (hereafter referred to as Compound 2), rhabdomyolysis was added to the product labelling about 10 years ago, and the cases upon which the decision to make the labelling change are currently held in a legacy database for which the adverse events have not been encoded using MedDRA. However, Compound 2 was the subject of a review for cases of rhabdomyolysis as part of a potential drug interaction about two years ago, and contains all cases for Compound 2 that had been reported for about the previous five years. The database was therefore reviewed for cases involving Compound 2 cases reporting events mapping to any of the PTs listed in the proposed SMQ through the cut-off date that was used for the review of possible drug interaction-related cases of rhabdomyolysis. For these two products, it was expected that the proposed search strategy would identify a reasonable pool of potential cases to be included in a case review.

Results

As a result of this review, a total of 49 relevant PTs were identified. The primary pathway for these 49 PTs has them listed under six SOCs, 12 High Level Group Terms (HLGTs), and 17 High Level Terms (HLTs).

Based on the PTs identified, queries of the database to identify relevant cases for review were conducted in a two-step manner. The first step was to conduct a "narrow" search to identify a "core" set of cases specifically reported to involve rhabdomyolysis, myopathy, or myopathy-related manifestations of muscle necrosis, myoglobinemia or myoglobinuria. This first search involved the nine rhabdomyolysis- or myopathy-related PTs listed in Table 1. In an effort to make this standard query relatively specific, not all possibly rhabdomyolysis- or myopathy-related events were included. For example, not all PTs listed under the HLT Myopathies are included. The other preferred terms under this HLT most likely refer to specific myopathy syndromes other than rhabdomyolysis that are not likely to be drug-related (such as Diabetic amyotrophy, Glycogen storage disease type V, and Myopathy endocrine) or are too drug specific (such as Myopathy steroid).

The second step was to conduct a "broad" search to identify cases that might be rhabdomyolysis or myopathy but were not specifically recognized as such at the time they were reported. Such rhabdomyolysis- or myopathy-like cases were identified by searching for cases not specifically reporting events that encode to any of the PTs listed in Table 1, but reporting events that encode to at least one of the 40 relevant PTs listed in Table 2.

The searches of Pfizer's early alert safety database using the proposed SMQ identified a total of 251 cases for Compound 1 and 318 cases for Compound 2. The results of these searches are summarized in Tables 3, 4, and 5. A listing of the number of cases reporting each of the relevant MedDRA PTs is presented in Table 3. The five most commonly reported PTs for both Compound 1 and Compound 2 were Myalgia, Blood creatine phosphokinase increased, Muscle weakness, Rhabdomyolysis, and Myopathy.

The number of cases identified by the narrow search and the number of cases added after the broad search is presented in Table 4. It should be noted that for Compound 1, the majority of cases were identified by the broad search, while for compound 2 the majority were identified by the narrow search.

In Table 5, the cases identified are further characterized by the presence of other PTs reported in the same case. Other than Rhabdomyolysis or Myopathy, the two most commonly reported PTs for both Compound 1 and Compound 2 were Myalgia (160 and 72 cases respectively) and Blood creatine phosphokinase increased (74 and 61 cases respectively). A number of cases for both test products reported both of these PTs in the same case, reported either Myalgia or Blood creatine phosphokinase increased along with another narrow or broad search PT or with a non-search PT that is often associated with rhabdomyolysis or myopathy (such as fever, fatigue, nausea, increased aminotransferases or lactic dehydrogenase). For purposes of this evaluation a case was considered to be a potential case of rhabdomyolysis or myopathy if it reported the PTs Rhabdomyolysis, Myopathy, or at least one other narrow PT; Myalgia, Myalgia aggravated, or Polymyalgia and Blood creatine phosphokinase increased; or any broad PT with at least one non-search PT associated with rhabdomyolysis or myopathy. Using these criteria, 73 (29%) of the 251 cases the proposed SMQ identified for Compound 1 and 247 (78%) of the 318 cases the proposed SMQ identified for Compound 2 would be considered potential cases of rhabdomyolysis or myopathy.

In the vast majority of the 178 cases for Compound 1 and 71 cases for Compound 2 that reported only one broad search PT, the SMQ search PT identified was the only reported adverse event term for the case. In these cases it is unlikely that the cases contain sufficient information to determine if the reported broad PTs were possibly the result of rhabdomyolysis or myopathy.

Summary and Conclusions

The MedDRA dictionary (version 5.1) was reviewed to identify search terms for inclusion in an SMQ to identify cases of potential rhabdomyolysis or myopathy. This review identified a total of 49 relevant PTs. The primary pathway for these 49 PTs has them listed under six SOCs, 12 HLGTs, and 17 HLTs. These 49 PTs can be divided into terms for inclusion in a narrow search to identify cases specifically reported to involve rhabdomyolysis and/or myopathy or myopathy-related manifestations such as muscle necrosis, myoglobinemia, or myoglobinuria, and a broad search to identify cases not specifically reported as rhabdomyolysis or myopathy but reporting other musculoskeletal, renal, metabolic, or laboratory PTs that might involve rhabdomyolysis or myopathy.

The SMQ was tested against two products, both of which had rhabdomyolysis added to the product labelling during their post-marketing experience.

The results of these tests indicate that the proposed SMQ satisfactorily identified an adequate pool of cases to be reviewed to determine if an association exists with rhabdomyolysis or myopathy for both of the test products. Based on these results, the proposed SMQ should be satisfactory for use to identify potential non-clinical study origin cases of rhabdomyolysis or myopathy reported during any drug product's post-marketing experience.

References

1 Basic requirements for the use of terms for reporting adverse drug reactions (IV). *Pharmacoepidemiology and Drug Safety* 1993; 2:149-153.

2 Myopathy. Reporting Adverse Drug Reactions: *Definitions of Terms and Criteria for Their Use.* Bankowski Z, Bruppacher R, Crusius I et al (Eds). Council for International Organizations of Medical Sciences: Geneva, 1999, pg. 16-17.

3 Poels PJE and Gabreëls FJM. Rhabdomyolysis: a review of the literature. *Clin Neurol Neurosurg* 1993; 95:175-192.

4 Omar MA, Wilson JP, and Cox, TS. Rhabdomyolysis and HMG-CoA reductase inhibitors. *Annals Pharmacother* 2001; 35:1096-1107.

5 Prendergast BD and George CF. Drug-induced rhabdomyolysis – mechanisms and management. *Postgrad Med J* 1993; 69:333-336.

MedDRA (version 5.1) Preferred Terms to Include for Rhabdomyolysis/Myopathy (Primary Pathways Sorted by SOC, HLGT, and HLT)

Table 1. Rhabdomyolysis- and Myopathy-Related Preferred Terms for Narrow Search

System Organ Class (SOC)	High Level Group Term (HLGT)	High Level Term (HLT)	Preferred Term (PT)
Musculoskeletal and connective tissue disorders	Muscle disorders	Myopathies	Muscle necrosis
			Myopathy
			Myopathy aggravated
			Myopathy toxic
			Rhabdomyolysis
		Muscle related signs and symptoms NEC	Myoglobinaemia
Renal and urinary abnormalities	Urinary tract signs and symptoms	Urinary abnormalities	Myoglobinuria
Investigations	Musculoskeletal and soft tissues investigations (excl enzyme tests)	Musculoskeletal and soft tissues tests NEC	Blood myoglobin increased
			Myoglobin urine present

MedDRA (version 5.1) Preferred Terms to Include for Rhabdomyolysis/Myopathy (Primary Pathways Sorted by SOC, HLGT, and HLT)

Table 2. Rhabdomyolysis- and Myopathy-Related Preferred Terms for Broad Search

System Organ Class (SOC)	High Level Group Term (HLGT)	High Level Term (HLT)	Preferred Term (PT)
Musculoskeletal and connective tissue disorders	Muscle disorders	Muscle related signs and symptoms NEC	Muscle haemorrhage
			Muscle fatigue
			Muscle disorder NOS
		Myopathies	Compartment syndrome
		Muscle pains	Myalgia
			Myalgia aggravated
			Myalgia intercostal
			Polymyalgia
			Polymyalgia aggravated
		Muscle weakness	Muscle weakness aggravated
			Muscle weakness NOS
	Musculoskeletal and connective tissue disorders NEC	Musculoskeletal and connective tissue signs and symptoms NEC	Musculoskeletal discomfort
			Musculoskeletal pain
			Musculoskeletal disorder NOS
Injury, poisoning and procedural complications	Injuries NEC	Muscle, tendon and ligament injuries	Muscle rupture
Investigations	Musculoskeletal and soft tissue investigations (excl enzyme tests)	Musculoskeletal and soft tissue histopathology procedures	Biopsy muscle abnormal
	Neurological and special senses investigations	Neurologic diagnostic procedures	Electromyogram abnormal
	Renal and urinary tract investigations and urinalyses	Renal function analyses	Blood creatinine abnormal
			Blood creatinine increased
			Creatinine renal clearance decreased
			Glomerular filtration rate abnormal

Table 2. Rhabdomyolysis- and Myopathy-Related Preferred Terms for Broad Search *(continued)*

System Organ Class (SOC)	High Level Group Term (HLGT)	High Level Term (HLT)	Preferred Term (PT)
			Glomerular filtration rate decreased
			Renal clearance NOS decreased
Investigations (Continued)	Enzyme investigations NEC	Skeletal and cardiac muscle analyses	Blood creatine phosphokinase abnormal NOS
			Blood creatine phosphokinase increased
			Blood creatine phosphokinase MM increased
			Muscle enzyme increased
	Water, electrolyte and mineral investigations	Mineral and electrolyte analyses	Blood calcium decreased
Renal and urinary disorders	Renal disorders (excl nephropathies)	Renal failure and impairment	Anuria
			Oliguria
			Progressive renal failure
			Renal failure acute
			Renal failure acute on chronic
			Renal failure aggravated
			Renal failure chronic aggravated
			Renal impairment NOS
		Renal vascular and ischaemic conditions	Renal tubular necrosis
	Urinary tract signs and symptoms	Urinary abnormalities	Chromaturia
Respiratory, thoracic and mediastinal disorders	Thoracic disorders (excl lung and pleura)	Diaphragmatic disorders (excl congenital)	Diaphragm muscle weakness
Metabolism and nutrition disorders	Bone, calcium, magnesium and phosphorus metabolism disorders	Calcium decreased disorders	Hypocalcaemia

Table 3. Health Care Professional, Non-Clinical Study Cases Reporting Rhabdomyolysis/Myopathy–Related MedDRA Preferred Terms for Two Test Products Reported to Pfizer's Early Alert Safety Database During the Time Periods Under Review

	Number of Cases	
MedDRA Preferred Term	Compound 1	Compound 2
Blood myoglobin increased *	—	1
Muscle necrosis *	—	5
Myoglobin urine present *	—	—
Myoglobinaemia *	—	—
Myoglobinuria *	—	3
Myopathy *	6	13
Myopathy aggravated *	—	—
Myopathy toxic *	—	—
Rhabdomyolysis *	14	189
Anuria †	—	—
Biopsy muscle abnormal †	—	—
Blood calcium decreased †	—	—
Blood creatine phosphokinase abnormal NOS †	—	—
Blood creatine phosphokinase increased †	74	61
Blood creatine phosphokinase MM increased †	—	—
Blood creatinine abnormal †	—	—
Blood creatinine increased †	—	8
Chromaturia †	4	7
Compartment syndrome †	—	—
Creatinine renal clearance decreased †	—	—
Diaphragm muscle weakness †	—	—
Electromyogram abnormal †	—	—
Glomerular filtration rate abnormal †	—	—
Glomerular filtration rate decreased †	—	—
Hypocalcaemia †	—	—
Muscle disorder NOS †	—	—
Muscle enzyme increased †	—	—
Muscle fatigue †	1	—
Muscle haemorrhage †	—	—
Muscle rupture †	—	—

(continued)

	Number of Cases	
MedDRA Preferred Term	**Compound 1**	**Compound 2**
Muscle weakness aggravated †	—	2
Muscle weakness NOS †	11	20
Musculoskeletal discomfort †	—	1
Musculoskeletal disorder NOS †	—	—
Musculoskeletal pain †	1	—
Myalgia †	160	72
Myalgia aggravated †	1	1
Myalgia intercostals †	—	—
Oliguria †	—	—
Polymyalgia †	1	—
Polymyalgia aggravated †	—	—
Progressive renal failure †	—	—
Renal clearance NOS decreased †	—	—
Renal failure acute †	1	13
Renal failure acute on chronic †	—	—
Renal failure aggravated †	—	—
Renal failure chronic aggravated †	—	—
Renal impairment NOS †	2	22
Renal tubular necrosis †	—	3
Total Cases Meeting Any SMQ Search Criteria	**251**	**318**
Total Health Care Professional Non-Clinical Study Cases	**1,716**	**822**

* event term for inclusion in narrow search
† event term for inclusion in broad search

Table 4. Number of Non-Clinical Study Cases Reported by Health Care Professionals Identified by Narrow and Broad Search for Rhabdomyolysis/Myopathy-Related Events

	Number of Cases Returned After Each Search	
Search Type	**Compound 1**	**Compound 2**
Narrow Search	30	213
Broad Search*	221	105
Total Cases Meeting Any SMQ Search Criteria	**251**	**318**
Total Health Care Professional Non-Clinical Study Cases	**1,716**	**822**

* cases reporting only broad search terms without reporting any narrow search terms

Table 5. Number of Non-Clinical Study Cases Reported by Health Care Professionals Identified by Search for Rhabdomyolysis/ Myopathy-Related Events Further Categorized by the Presence of Other Preferred Terms Reported in the Same Case

	Number of Cases	
Search PTs Categorized by Presence of Other Reported PTs	**Compound 1**	**Compound 2**
Rhabdomyolysis and/or Myopathy	20	201
Myalgia, Myalgia aggravated, or Polymyalgia and Blood creatine phosphokinase increased	17	21
Myalgia, Myalgia aggravated, or Polymyalgia with at least one narrow PT other than Rhabdomyolysis or Myopathy	2	3
Myalgia, Myalgia aggravated, or Polymyalgia with at least one additional broad PT*	1	—
Blood creatine phosphokinase increased with at least one narrow PT other than Rhabdomyolysis or Myopathy	—	4
Blood creatine phosphokinase increased with at least one additional broad PT†	—	1
Myalgia, Myalgia aggravated, or Polymyalgia with at least one non-search PT associated with rhabdomyolysis or myopathy	17	3
Blood creatine phosphokinase increased with at least one non-search PT associated with rhabdomyolysis or myopathy	6	2
Other narrow PT with at least one other broad PT	—	2
Other narrow PTs with at least one non-search PT associated with rhabdomyolysis or myopathy	2	3
Other narrow PTs only relevant PT	8	7
Total Cases of Potential Rhabdomyolysis or Myopathy‡	**73**	**247**
Myalgia, Myalgia aggravated, or Polymyalgia only relevant PT	122	40
Blood creatine phosphokinase increased only relevant PT	49	26

(continued)

Search PTs Categorized by Presence of Other Reported PTs	Number of Cases	
	Compound 1	Compound 2
Other broad PTs only relevant PT	7	5
Total Cases Reporting Only One Broad PT	**178**	**71**
Total Cases Meeting Any SMQ Search Criteria	**251**	**318**

* at least one additional broad PT other than Blood creatine phosphokinase increased

† at least one additional broad PT other than Myalgia, Myalgia aggravated, or Polymyalgia.

‡ any case reporting Rhabdomyolysis, Myopathy, or ≥1 other narrow PT; Myalgia, Myalgia aggravated, or Polymyalgia and Blood creatine phosphokinase increased; or any broad PT with ≥1 non-search term associated with rhabdomyolysis/myopathy considered a potential case of rhabdomyolysis or myopathy.

VI. Examples of Candidate SMQs

Hepatic Disorders

**This SMQ is not for routine use.
It Is only an example.**

1. Introduction

The Standardised MedDRA Query (SMQ) on Hepatic Disorders is relatively complicated since it concerns events which relate to a whole organ system.

It comprises

- **A comprehensive search of all terms possibly related to the liver, irrespective whether they are possible related to drug effects**
- **A number of sub-searches on some specific liver related topics**
- **Searches for terms for potentially drug related liver disorders.**

MedDRA terms related to the liver

Terms concerning hepatic disorders and related conditions are present in 12 of the MedDRA System Organ Classes (SOCs): Hepatobiliary Disorders, Investigations, Neoplasms benign, malignant and unspecified (incl cysts and polyps), Congenital, familial and genetic disorders, Infections and infestations, Nervous system disorders, Metabolism and nutrition disorders, Gastrointestinal disorders, General disorders and administration site conditions, Respiratory, thoracic and mediastinal disorders, Surgical and medical procedures, Skin and subcutaneous tissue disorders.

2. Search Strategy

There are three types of searches

- **Search 1: This is a comprehensive SMQ on all types of liver related events**. It contains all hepatic disorder terms from all of the the above mentioned 12 MedDRA SOCs and therefore retrieves all cases with liver related conditions irrespective of whether they relate to drug-induced disorders, medical history, congenital disorders etc.

This is a very broad general search on all hepatic disorders including neoplasms, infections and congenital disorders. It retrieves all cases, which are in any way related to the liver and includes all terms of the sub-searches 2.1- 2.11.

- **Search 2: This SMQ comprises 11 sub-searches (2.1 to 2.11)** retrieving all cases concerning one of 11 liver related specific topics. This permits searches concerning specific liver related topics. Depending on the issue in many cases a combination of several of these sub-searches is appropriate. Please note that the sub-searches are not mutually exclusive which must be taken into account when using combinations of several sub-searches. Since single cases may contain a number of different terms included in different sub-searches a given case may be retrieved in more that one sub-search if not a combined "hit list" is used for the retrieval.
- **Search 3: This SMQ** comprises two search combinations (3.1 and 3.2) for potentially drug related liver disorder, a comprehensive search (3.1) and one limited to severe (often serious) events (3.2).

General remarks

This SMQ on Hepatic Disorders only lists terms linking to primary SOCs but many terms of other SOCs also have secondary links to the SOC Hepatobiliary Disorders.

Not included in this SMQ are terms solely associated to disorders of the **gallbladder** and the **bile duct**.

It may be helpful in some instances to start with the **full general search excluding one or more of the specific sub-searches** in order to eliminate conditions which are not applicable for a given question such as liver infections (sub-search 2.9) or congenital and neonatal conditions (sub-search 2.7).

The term **Hepatitis** is frequently misused in adverse reaction reporting by referring to any liver damage, whether or not histological lesions have been confirmed. This problem can, of course, not be solved by any SMQ and requires an analysis of narratives and laboratory data fields.

Listing of the Searches provided:

Search 1	**Hepatic disorders – General search** Contains all terms of all sub-searches 2.1 to 2.11
Search 2	**Sub-searches on specific liver related topics**
Sub-search 2.1	Liver related investigations, signs and symptoms
Sub-search 2.2	Cholestasis and jaundice of hepatic origin
Sub-search 2.3	Hepatitis non-infectious
Sub-search 2.4	Liver neoplasms malignant and unspecified
Sub-search 2.5	Liver neoplasms benign
Sub-search 2.6	Hepatic failure, fibrosis and cirrhosis and other liver damage related conditions
Sub-search 2.7	Congenital, familial, neonatal and genetic disorders of the liver
Sub-search 2.8	Possibly liver related coagulation and bleeding disturbances
Sub-search 2.9	Liver infections
Sub-search 2.10	Events specifically reported as alcohol related
Sub-search 2.11	Pregnancy related hepatic disorders
Search 3	**Searches for possibly drug related hepatic disorders** Based on combinations of sub-searches 2.1 to 2.11
Sub-search 3.1	Possibly drug related hepatic disorders – Comprehensive search
Sub-search 3.2	Possibly drug related hepatic disorders – Severe events only

3. Specifications

All MedDRA terms which are used in the present version of this document are from MedDRA version 6.1.

Search 1 Hepatic disorders – General search

To be used for a general search retrieving all types of hepatic disorders. It combines all of the terms of the sub-searches 2.1 to 2.11.

Search 2 Sub-searches on specific liver related topics

Sub-search 2.1 Liver related investigations, signs and symptoms

Most of the terms of this sub-search belong to the HLGT Hepatobiliary investigations of the SOC Investigations. Many terms of this HLGT, however, relate to investigations as such (without indicating a result) or to investigations with a normal outcome; these terms are not included in this search. In addition this search contains all terms of the HLT Hepatobiliary signs and symptoms of the SOC Hepatobiliary disorders and a few PT of other SOCs.

Included are:

- The following PT of to the HLT Liver function analyses: Alanine aminotransferase abnormal, Alanine aminotransferase increased, Ammonia abnormal, Ammonia increased, Aspartate aminotransferase abnormal, Aspartate aminotransferase increased, Bile output abnormal, Bile output decreased, Bilirubin conjugated increased, Blood bilirubin abnormal, Blood bilirubin increased, Blood bilirubin unconjugated increased, Blood cholinesterase abnormal, Blood cholinesterase decreased, Bromosulphthalein test abnormal, Galactose elimination capacity test abnormal, Galactose elimination capacity test decreased, Gamma-glutamyltransferase abnormal, Gamma-glutamyltransferase increased, Guanase increased, Hepaplastin abnormal, Hepaplastin decreased, Hepatic enzyme decreased, Hepatic enzyme increased, Hepatic enzyme abnormal, Hyperammonaemia, Leucine aminopeptidase increased, Liver function test abnormal, Retinol binding protein decreased, Transaminases abnormal, Transaminases increased, Urine bilirubin increased, Urobilin urine present, 5'nucleotidase increased.
- The following PT of the HLT Hepatobiliary histopathology procedures: Biopsy liver abnormal.
- The following PT of the HLT Hepatobiliary imaging procedures: Liver scan abnormal, Ultrasound liver abnormal, X-ray hepatobiliary abnormal.
- The following PT of the HLT Tissue enzyme analyses NEC: Blood alkaline phosphatase increased, Blood alkaline phosphatase abnormal.
- The following PT of the HLT Hepatic enzyme and function abnormalities: Hepatic function abnormal

- The following PT of the HLT Hepatobiliary signs and symptoms: Caput medusae, Foetor hepaticus, Hepatic congestion, Hepatic pain, Hepatomegaly, Hepatosplenomegaly, Liver induration, Liver tenderness, Perihepatic discomfort.
- The following PT of the HLT Hepatobiliary disorders NEC: Hypercholia
- The following additional PT Ascites, Haemorrhagic ascites, Kayser-Fleischer ring, Hyperbilirubinaemia, Hypoalbuminaemia, Liver palpable subcostal, Hepatic mass.
- The PT Oedema due to hepatic disease of the SOC General disorders and administration site conditions

Sub-search 2.2 Cholestasis and Jaundice of hepatic origin

This search includes all conditions associated with jaundice or cholestasis of possible hepatic origin and therefore excludes PTs indicating jaundice caused by haemolytic conditions, the PT Jaundice extrahepatic obstructive and the LLT Hemorrhagic leptospirosis with jaundice.

Included are:

- SOC Hepatobiliary disorders
  - HLT Cholestasis and jaundice: The PT Cholestasis, Hepatitis cholestatic. Hyperbilirubinaemia, Jaundice cholestatic, Jaundice Hepatocellular, Jaundice.
  - HLT Hepatobiliary disorders NEC: The PT Cholaemia
  - HLT Hepatic enzymes and function abnormalities: The PT Bilirubin excretion disorder
- SOC Eye disorders: The PT Ocular icterus.
- SOC Investigations - HLT Liver function analyses: The PT Icterus index increased.

Sub-search 2.3 Hepatitis non-infectious

Included are of the SOC Hepatobiliary disorders

- The following PT of the HLT Hepatocellular damage and hepatitis NEC: Autoimmune hepatitis, Chronic hepatitis, Cytolytic hepatitis, Hepatitis acute, Hepatitis chronic active, Hepatitis chronic persistent, Hepatitis fulminant, Hepatitis granulomatous, Hepatitis, Hepatitis toxic, Ischaemic hepatitis, Non-alcoholic steatohepatitis. (The remaining PT of this HLT are included in searches 2.7 and 2.11)
- The PT Hepatitis cholestatic of the HLT Cholestasis and jaundice.
- The PT Radiation hepatitis of the HLT Radiation injuries.

Sub-search 2.4 Liver neoplasms malignant and unspecified

All terms of this search belong to the HLGT Hepatobiliary neoplasms malignant and unspecified of the SOC Neoplasms benign, malignant and unspecified (incl cysts and polyps).

Included are

- All PT of the HLT Hepatic neoplasms malignant: Hepatic cancer metastatic, Hepatic cancer stage I, Hepatic cancer stage II, Hepatic cancer stage III, Hepatic cancer stage IV, Hepatic neoplasm malignant non-resectable, Hepatic neoplasm malignant, Hepatic neoplasm malignant recurrent, Hepatic neoplasm malignant resectable, Liver carcinoma ruptured.
- Both PT of the HLT Hepatoblastomas: Hepatoblastoma, Hepatoblastoma recurrent.
- The following PT of the HLT Hepatobiliary neoplasms malignant NEC: Hepatobiliary carcinoma in situ, Malignant hepatobiliary neoplasm, Mixed hepatocellular cholangiocarcinoma.
- The following PT of the HLT Hepatobiliary neoplasms malignancy unspecified: PT Hepatic neoplasm, Hepatobiliary neoplasm.

Sub-search 2.5 Liver Neoplasms Benign

All terms of this search belong to the SOC Neoplasms benign, malignant and unspecified (incl cysts and polyps).

Included are of the HLGT Hepatic and biliary neoplasms benign

- The following PT of the HLT Hepatobiliary neoplasms benign: Benign hepatic neoplasm, Focal nodular hyperplasia, Haemangioma of liver, Hepatic adenoma, Hepatic cyst, Hepatic cyst ruptured, Hepatic haemangioma rupture

Sub-search 2.6 Hepatic failure, fibrosis and cirrhosis and other liver damage related conditions

This search is as a rule not used alone but in combination with sub-search 2.3 - Hepatitis non-infectious. The search does not include the PT Cardiac cirrhosis which is secondary to a cardiac condition.

Included are

- SOC Hepatobiliary disorders
  - All PT of the HLT Hepatic failure and associated disorders: Hepatic failure, Hepatorenal failure, Hepatorenal syndrome.
  - The following PT of the HLT Hepatic fibrosis and cirrhosis: PT Biliary cirrhosis, Hepatic cirrhosis, Biliary cirrhosis primary,

Lupoid hepatic cirrhosis, Hepatic fibrosis, Biliary fibrosis, Nodular regenerative hyperplasia (PT Cirrhosis alcoholic is included in search 2.10 PT Congenital hepatic fibrosis is included in search 2.7)

  - The following PT of the HLT Hepatocellular damage and hepatitis NEC: Hepatic necrosis, Hepatic steatosis, Hepatocellular damage, Hepatocellular foamy cell syndrome, Hepatotoxicity, Non-alcoholic steatohepatitis, Portal triaditis, Reye's syndrome.
  - The following PT of the HLT Hepatic and hepatobiliary disorders NEC: Hepatobiliary disease, Liver disorder, Hepatic lesion, Hepatic atrophy.
  - The PT Portal hypertension of the HLT Hepatic vascular disorders.
- SOC Nervous system disorders
  - PT Asterixis, Coma hepatic and Hepatic encephalopathy
- SOC Gastrointestinal disorders
  - PT Ascites, Varices oesophageal, Oesophageal varices haemorrhage.
- SOC Skin and subcutaneous tissue disorders
  - PT Spider naevus.
- SOC Respiratory, thoracic and mediastinal disorders
  - PT Hepatopulmonary syndrome
- SOC Surgical and medical procedures
  - PT Liver transplant, PT Liver and small intestine transplant, PT Renal and liver transplant, PT Hepatectomy, PT Liver operation.
- SOC General disorders and administration site conditions
  - PT Oedema due to hepatic disease

Sub-search 2.7 Congenital, familial, neonatal and genetic disorders of the liver

Included are

- SOC Congenital, familial and genetic disorders
  - The following PT of the HLT Hepatobiliary abnormalities congenital: Accessory liver lobe, Alagille syndrome, Congenital absence of bile ducts, Congenital cystic disease of liver, Congenital hepatic fibrosis, Congenital hepatobiliary anomaly, Congenital hepatomegaly, Dilatation intrahepatic duct congenital, Hereditary haemochromatosis, Polycystic liver disease.

- The following PT with a secondary link to the HLT Hepatic metabolic disorders: Porphyria acute, Porphyria non-acute, Pseudoporphyria, Hepato-lenticular degeneration
- The following PT with a secondary link to the HLT Hepatic and hepatobiliary disorders NEC: Cerebrohepatorenal syndrome.
- The following PT related to neonatal conditions: Hepato-splenomegaly neonatal, Neonatal hepatomegaly, Hyperbilirubinaemia neonatal, Neonatal cholestasis, Jaundice neonatal, Kernicterus, Hepatitis neonatal, Hepatocellular damage neonatal.

Sub-search 2.8 Possibly liver related coagulation and bleeding disturbances

This search includes decreases of coagulation factor levels which may be due to reduced liver function and changes in blood coagulation parameters depending on these factors.

Included are of the SOC Investigations

- The following PT of the HLT Coagulation and bleeding analyses: Antithrombin III decreased, Blood fibrinogen abnormal, Blood fibrinogen decreased, Blood thrombin abnormal, Blood thrombin decreased, Blood thromboplastin abnormal, Blood thromboplastin decreased, Coagulation factor decreased, Coagulation factor IX level abnormal, Coagulation factor IX level decreased, Coagulation factor V level abnormal, Coagulation factor V level decreased, Coagulation factor VII level abnormal, Coagulation factor VII level decreased, Coagulation factor X level abnormal, Coagulation factor X level decreased, International normalised ratio abnormal, International normalised ratio decreased, Protein C decreased, Protein S abnormal, Protein S decreased, Prothrombin level abnormal, Prothrombin level decreased, Prothrombin time abnormal, Prothrombin time prolonged, Prothrombin time ratio abnormal, Prothrombin time ratio decreased, Thrombin time abnormal, Thrombin time prolonged.

Sub-search 2.9 Liver infections

Included are

- SOC Infections and infestations
  - All PT of the HLT Hepatitis viral infections: Hepatitis A, Hepatitis B, Hepatitis C, Hepatitis D, Hepatitis E, Hepatitis F, Hepatitis G, Hepatitis H, Hepatitis non-A non-B, Hepatitis non-A non-B non-C, Gianotti-Crosti syndrome.

- The following PT of the HLT Liver and spleen infections: Hepatobiliary infection, Hepatic infection, Hepatic cyst infection, Liver abscess, Portal pyaemia (not included are splenic infections).
- The following PT linking to various infection related HLT: Hepatitis infectious mononucleosis, Hepatitis viral, Cytomegalovirus hepatitis, Hepatitis syphilitic, Hepatitis toxoplasmal, Hepatitis mumps, Hepatitis infectious, Viral hepatitis carrier, Adenoviral hepatitis, Hepatic candidiasis, Hepatosplenic candidiasis, Amoebic liver abscess, Hepatic echinococciasis, Schistosomiasis liver, Perihepatitis gonococcal, Weil's disease.

– SOC Hepatobiliary disorders:
  - The following PT of the HLT Hepatic viral infections: Hepatitis post transfusion
– SOC Congenital, familial and genetic disorders
  - The PT Congenital hepatitis B infection
– SOC Investigations
  - The following PT: Anti-HBc antibody positive, Anti-HBe antibody positive, Anti-HBs antibody positive, Anti-HBc IgM antibody positive, Anti-HBc IgG antibody positive, Hepatitis A antibody positive, Hepatitis A positive, Hepatitis A antigen positive, Hepatitis A antibody abnormal, Hepatitis B positive, Hepatitis B antibody abnormal, Hepatitis B antibody positive, Hepatitis B DNA assay positive, Hepatitis B surface antigen positive, Hepatitis B core antigen positive, Hepatitis B e antigen positive, Hepatitis C antibody positive, Hepatitis C positive, Hepatitis C RNA positive, Hepatitis D antibody positive, Hepatitis D antigen positive, Hepatitis D RNA positive, Hepatitis E antibody abnormal, Hepatitis E antibody positive, Hepatitis E antigen positive.

The following PT of the SOC Investigations are not included in this search: Hepatitis A virus, Hepatitis A screen, Hepatitis A antibody, Hepatitis A antigen normal, Hepatitis B virus, Hepatitis B antibody normal, Hepatitis B antibody negative, Hepatitis B antibody, Hepatitis B surface antigen negative, Hepatitis B surface antigen, Hepatitis B screen, Hepatitis B core antigen, Hepatitis B e antigen negative, Hepatitis B e antigen, Hepatitis B virus, Hepatitis C virus, Hepatitis C antibody, Hepatitis C antibody negative, Hepatitis C RNA, Hepatitis C RNA negative, Hepatitis C screen, Hepatitis D antigen, Hepatitis D antigen negative, Hepatitis E antibody, Hepatitis E antibody normal, Hepatitis E antibody negative, Hepatitis viral test.

Sub-search 2.10 Events specifically reported as alcohol related

This search contains terms specifically related to alcohol associated disorders. These have not been included in any of the other sub-searches since alcohol related terms are normally not searched for when looking for drug induced liver injuries. Possibly alcohol related events which also can have other caused (e.g. cirrhosis) have not been included here.

Included are

- PT Alcoholic liver disease, Cirrhosis alcoholic, Fatty liver alcoholic, Hepatitis alcoholic, Zieve syndrome

Sub-search 2.11 Pregnancy related hepatic disorders

This search contains terms specifically related to pregnancy associated disorders. These have not been included in any of the other sub-searches since they are normally not searched for when looking for drug induced liver injuries.

Included are

- PT Cholestasis of pregnancy, Acute fatty liver of pregnancy.

Search 3 Searches for possibly drug related hepatic disorders

Sub-search 3.1 Possibly drug related hepatic disorders – Comprehensive search

Searches 3.1 and 3.2 provide combinations of the searches 2.1 to 2.11 for terms associated with possibly drug related hepatic disorders.

This Broad search includes all terms from the following searches:

- Sub-search 2.1 Liver related investigations, signs and symptoms
- Sub-search 2.2 Cholestasis and Jaundice of hepatic origin
- Sub-search 2.3 Hepatitis non-infectious
- Sub-search 2.4 Liver neoplasms malignant and unspecified
- Sub-search 2.5 Liver neoplasms benign
- Sub-search 2.6 Hepatic failure, fibrosis and cirrhosis and other liver related conditions
- Sub-search 2.8 Possibly liver related coagulation and bleeding disorders

Sub-search 3.2 Possibly drug related hepatic disorders – Severe events only

This search for severe, often serious reactions includes all terms from the following searches:

- Sub-search 2.3 Hepatitis non-infectious
- Sub-search 2.4 Liver neoplasms malignant and unspecified
- Sub-search 2.5 Liver Neoplasms Benign
- Sub-search 2.6 Hepatic failure, fibrosis and cirrhosis and other liver damage related conditions

4. Pre-release testing

The most important requirement for the quality of an SMQ is whether it contains all of the MedDRA terms to which cases relevant for the given question are coded. It is also important to avoid as far as possible non-specific terms which when reported alone without other more specific terms are not suggestive of relevant cases for the topic concerned and thus increase background noise.

For the SMQs on Hepatic Disorders three approaches were chosen as follows.

4.1 Completeness of data – based on BfArM database

Current situation at BfArM

For the purpose of coding adverse reactions WHO-ART is the terminology currently used at BfArM. MedRA-implementation is scheduled for mid 2004. Therefore, the test cannot be run on the data directly; it is necessary to convert the data to be accessable with the MedDRA-terminology.

Conversion of data

The codeplan consists of about 5700 German terms, that are considered as either translations of (4000) or assignments to (1700) terms of the original terminology. The German terms that were used for coding of the ADR are is stored in the database in addition to the WHO-ART preferred term. ADR descriptions not reflected in WHO-ART are maintained as verbatims in the database.

The conversion to MedDRA 6.0 has been done as follows: The links between the German terms and MedDRA have been created on the basis of LLTs. Since MedDRA PTs are also LLTs we could make use of the existing German PT translations for an assignment on LLT-level. The conversion has been done in four steps:

1. German Terms with an exact string match to a German MedDRA PT/LLT. No further review was considered necessary.

2. German Terms with no exact string match to MedDRA but which are considered translations of WHO-ART-terms as published on our website were linked to LLTs according to the respective WHO-ART record-number if included in MedDRA.
3. Remaining German Terms of our catalogue were reviewed and assigned to MedDRA LLTs on a term by term basis.
4. Verbatim terms that have not been coded in WHO-ART so far were also reviewed term by term and linked to MedDRA LLTs where possible

For the purpose of this SMQ testing, all relevant terms could be matched with MedDRA.

Test of SMQ "Hepatic Disorders"

Unlike other SMQs the SMQ for hepatic disorders aims to include all liver-related terms and to reorder them in different sub-searches. Therefore, it can be anticipated that all cases describing liver related conditions will be detected when using the sub-searches alone or in combination. The test focussed to detect potential terms which were not yet covered in one of these sub-searches.

For the purpose of this test case reports from Germany since 1995 were considered (approximately 89000). The SMQ-PTs (all categories) were linked to database terms using the matches and assignments described above. Terms linked to one of the sub-searches were considered "covered". All others were grouped and reviewed on LLT-level (about 7000) for potential relevance to this SMQ. The test showed that there were no additional terms necessary to be included.

4.2 Testing on a company database (A)

Methods

In an effort to determine how well the proposed searches 3.1 and 3.2 of the SMQ for liver disorders would identify potential cases of possibly drug induced liver toxicity, the company drug safety database was searched using the proposed search strategies. MedDRA version 6.1 is currently used to code cases. The database contains cases of adverse events (serious and non-serious) reported spontaneously, including cases reported from health authorities and cases published in the medical literature. It also contains cases of serious adverse events reported from clinical studies and company-sponsored marketing programs regardless of causality. It was reviewed for cases reported through 18 February 2004 that contain a MedDRA PT belonging to search 3.1 and /or 3.2 (adverse event or comanifestation) for four different drugs. Liver toxicity is attributed to two of the four drugs (hereafter referred to as Compound 1 and Compound 2) and is addressed in the company core data sheet (CDS) for these two products. The remaining two products (hereafter referred to as Compound 3 and Compound 4), are not currently thought to be associated with liver toxicity.

Results and Discussion

As a result of applying the two searches for possibly drug induced hepatotoxicity to the data of the four test drug in the database, a total of 32 PTs belonging to search 3.2 (which focuses on possibly severe events), were identified (see table 1). In addition, another 38 PTs that are not already contained in search 3.2 were retrieved with the broader search 3.1.

The results of the search for the four test compounds are summarized in Tables 1 and 2. In both tables bold figures indicate that the percentage of of cases for a PT is higher for the test compound than for all remaining drugs on the database (data for remaining drugs is not shown). A case having an adverse event/comanifestation belonging to search 3.2 can additionally also contain another event/comanifestation belonging to search 3.1. It is also possible that a case contains more than one PT belonging to a sub-search. In Table 1, where PTs are displayed on an event/comanifestation level, such a case can be counted more than once. On the other hand in table 2, a case is counted only once, because the data is displayed at a case level.

A listing of the number of each of the relevant MedDRA PTs reported with the four drugs is presented in Table 1. The number of cases identified by the search for severe events (search 3.2) and the number of cases added after the broad search (search 3.1) is presented in Table 2. As the number of reports with each of the four compounds is quite different, percentages (number of reports of a certain PT belonging to the search reported with the drug in question compared to the number of events entered in the database with the drug in question in total) are also provided, to ease the interpretation of the findings. Furthermore, the percentage figures of a PT reported with the four test compounds were compared to the percentage figure of that PT reported with all remaining drugs entered on the database (327'270 cases), and percentages with a higher frequency on a test drug compared to the remaining drugs are bolded.

As can be seen from table 2, for the two products known to be associated with liver toxicity (Compounds 1 and 2), more than 10% of the total cases reported with each of these two drugs contain a PT belonging to search 3.1 or 3.2. This is considerably more than with the other two drugs (Compounds 3 and 4) where it is 1.5% and 3.7% respectively. As expected, compared to Compounds 3 and 4, the two compounds with known hepatotoxicity (Compound 1 and 2) both have a higher percentage of events belonging to search 3.2 (1.5% and 3.6% versus 0.4% and 1.9%) and search 3.1 (11.0% and 6.4% versus 1.1% and 2.1%).

Thus, for drug products clearly associated with liver toxicity, the proposed searches 3.1 and 3.2 seems to adequately identified cases of possible liver toxicity.

Summary and Conclusions

Searches 3.1 and 3.2 of the liver SMQ, which were both specifically designed to identify possibly drug-induced liver toxicity, were tested in the ADVENT database against four Roche drugs. Liver toxicity is attributed to two of the four drugs and the remaining two drugs are not currently thought to be associated with liver toxicity. The results of these tests indicate that the proposed two specific searches 3.1 and 3.2 seem to identify cases of drugs associated with liver toxicity, i.e. these two searches are an adequate tool to retrieve possibly relevant cases to assess if a drug has a hepatotoxic potential.

4.3 Testing on a company database (B)

A complementary analysis was used on the database of company B which is also coded using MedDRA version 6.1. Five drugs were analysed, two with known liver toxicity (A, B) and three with no known liver toxicity (C, D, E). For all of the sub-searches 2.1 to 2.11 odds ratios were calculated compared to the relative occurrence for the given term in the whole database.

The table shows the odds ratios for the percentage of events retrieved for the five drugs compared to that of all drugs available in the whole database for those sub-searches relevant for potential drug-related liver disorders.

Sub-search		Drug				
		A	B	C	D	E
1	General search	4.0	1.4	0.8	0.3	0.6
2.1	Liver related investigations, signs and symptoms	4.8	1.7	1.0	0.3	0.6
2.2	Cholestasis and jaundice of hepatic origin	2.6	1.1	0.3	0.2	0.6
2.3	Hepatitis non-infectious	3.1	0.7	0.4	0.2	0.8
2.6	Hepatic failure, fibrosis and cirrhosis and other liver damage related conditions	2.9	3.2	0.4	0.2	0.1
2.8	Coagulation and bleeding	1.9	1.3	0.2	0.3	0.5
3.1	Possibly drug related – Broad	4.0	1.4	0.8	0.3	0.6
3.2	Possibly drug related – Severe only	3.0	2.0	0.4	0.3	0.4

The data show that for all drugs for which no liver related events are listed in the CDS (C, D, E) the odds ratio was £ 1 for all of the sub-searches whereas for drugs A and B is was Δ 1 for all of them except search 2.3 for drug B. The odds ratios for drug B were for most sub-searches lower than for drug A which in accordance with current knowledge about these drugs.

Table 1. Adverse event and comanifestation PTs belonging to the searches for possible drug induced liver toxicity for four test products entered onto Roche's Drug Safety Database ADVENT through 19 February 2004

MedDRA Preferred Terms	Sub-search	Search 3.1	Search 3.2	Compound 1		Compound 2		Compound 3		Compound 4	
				N	%	N	%	N	%	N	%
SMQ Search 3.2 (Only severe possibly drug induced hepatic events)											
Autoimmune hepatitis	2.3	Y	Y	0	0.000%	0	0.000%	2	0.004%	0	0.000%
Cytolytic hepatitis	2.3	Y	Y	0	0.000%	12	0.049%	2	0.004%	1	0.008%
Hepatitis	2.3	Y	Y	8	0.186%	143	0.578%	35	0.070%	21	0.170%
Hepatitis acute	2.3	Y	Y	1	0.023%	3	0.012%	1	0.002%	0	0.000%
Hepatitis cholestatic	2.3	Y	Y	0	0.000%	73	0.295%	6	0.012%	5	0.041%
Hepatitis chronic active	2.3	Y	Y	0	0.000%	2	0.008%	0	0.000%	1	0.008%
Hepatitis fulminant	2.3	Y	Y	3	0.070%	4	0.016%	1	0.002%	1	0.008%
Hepatitis granulomatous	2.3	Y	Y	0	0.000%	4	0.016%	0	0.000%	0	0.000%
Hepatitis toxic	2.3	Y	Y	1	0.023%	15	0.061%	2	0.004%	1	0.008%
Total number of events in sub-search 2.3	**2.3**			**13**	**0.303%**	**256**	**1.035%**	**49**	**0.098%**	**30**	**0.243%**
Hepatic neoplasm	2.4	Y	Y	1	0.023%	1	0.004%	0	0.000%	0	0.000%
Hepatic neoplasm malignant	2.4	Y	Y	1	0.023%	0	0.000%	4	0.008%	1	0.008%
Malignant hepatobiliary neoplasm	2.4	Y	Y	1	0.023%	0	0.000%	1	0.002%	0	0.000%
Total number of events in sub-search 2.4	**2.4**			**3**	**0.070%**	**1**	**0.004%**	**5**	**0.010%**	**1**	**0.008%**
Hepatic cyst	2.5	Y	Y	2	0.047%	0	0.000%	1	0.002%	0	0.000%
Total number of events in sub-search 2.5	**2.5**			**2**	**0.047%**	**0**	**0.000%**	**1**	**0.002%**	**0**	**0.000%**

(continued)

MedDRA Preferred Terms	Sub-search	Search 3.1	Search 3.2	Compound 1		Compound 2		Compound 3		Compound 4	
				N	%	N	%	N	%	N	%
Ascites	2.6	Y	Y	4	0.093%	14	0.057%	5	0.010%	1	0.008%
Biliary cirrhosis	2.6	Y	Y	0	0.000%	0	0.000%	0	0.000%	1	0.008%
Coma hepatic	2.6	Y	Y	1	0.023%	1	0.004%	0	0.000%	2	0.016%
Hepatic atrophy	2.6	Y	Y	0	0.000%	0	0.000%	1	0.002%	0	0.000%
Hepatic cirrhosis	2.6	Y	Y	1	0.023%	3	0.012%	3	0.006%	3	0.024%
Hepatic encephalopathy	2.6	Y	Y	2	0.047%	6	0.024%	0	0.000%	1	0.008%
Hepatic failure	2.6	Y	Y	1	0.023%	32	0.129%	6	0.012%	4	0.032%
Hepatic fibrosis	2.6	Y	Y	0	0.000%	0	0.000%	0	0.000%	1	0.008%
Hepatic necrosis	2.6	Y	Y	3	0.070%	16	0.065%	2	0.004%	3	0.024%
Hepatic steatosis	2.6	Y	Y	3	0.070%	10	0.040%	21	0.042%	2	0.016%
Hepatocellular damage	2.6	Y	Y	0	0.000%	42	0.170%	6	0.012%	8	0.065%
Hepatorenal failure	2.6	Y	Y	0	0.000%	2	0.008%	0	0.000%	1	0.008%
Hepatorenal syndrome	2.6	Y	Y	0	0.000%	4	0.016%	0	0.000%	0	0.000%
Hepatotoxicity	2.6	Y	Y	0	0.000%	8	0.032%	1	0.002%	0	0.000%
Liver disorder	2.6	Y	Y	0	0.000%	24	0.097%	13	0.026%	6	0.049%
Oesophageal varices haemorrhage	2.6	Y	Y	0	0.000%	1	0.004%	0	0.000%	0	0.000%
Portal hypertension	2.6	Y	Y	0	0.000%	0	0.000%	1	0.002%	0	0.000%
Reye's syndrome	2.6	Y	Y	0	0.000%	2	0.008%	0	0.000%	0	0.000%
Varices oesophageal	2.6	Y	Y	0	0.000%	0	0.000%	1	0.002%	0	0.000%
Total number of events in sub-search 2.6	**2.6**			**15**	**0.350%**	**165**	**0.667%**	**60**	**0.120%**	**33**	**0.267%**

MedDRA Preferred Terms	Sub-search	Search 3.1	Search 3.2	Compound 1		Compound 2		Compound 3		Compound 4	
				N	%	N	%	N	%	N	%
SMQ Search 3.1 (Broad Drug induced hepatotoxicity search)*											
Alanine aminotransferase abnormal	2.1	Y		0	0.000%	0	0.000%	2	0.004%	0	0.000%
Alanine aminotransferase increased	2.1	Y		55	1.282%	105	0.424%	55	0.110%	25	0.203%
Ammonia increased	2.1	Y		1	0.023%	0	0.000%	0	0.000%	1	0.008%
Aspartate aminotransferase abnormal	2.1	Y		0	0.000%	0	0.000%	1	0.002%	0	0.000%
Aspartate aminotransferase increased	2.1	Y		57	1.328%	109	0.441%	48	0.096%	24	0.195%
Bilirubin conjugated increased	2.1	Y		3	0.070%	0	0.000%	2	0.004%	0	0.000%
Biopsy liver abnormal	2.1	Y		0	0.000%	1	0.004%	0	0.000%	0	0.000%
Blood alkaline phosphatase abnormal	2.1	Y		0	0.000%	1	0.004%	0	0.000%	0	0.000%
Blood alkaline phosphatase increased	2.1	Y		58	1.352%	108	0.437%	27	0.054%	14	0.113%
Blood bilirubin abnormal	2.1	Y		0	0.000%	0	0.000%	1	0.002%	0	0.000%
Blood bilirubin increased	2.1	Y		39	0.909%	71	0.287%	17	0.034%	12	0.097%
Blood cholinesterase decreased	2.1	Y		0	0.000%	0	0.000%	1	0.002%	0	0.000%
Gamma-glutamyltransferase abnormal	2.1	Y		4	0.093%	0	0.000%	1	0.002%	0	0.000%
Gamma-glutamyltransferase increased	2.1	Y		38	0.886%	55	0.222%	48	0.096%	20	0.162%
Hepatic congestion	2.1	Y		0	0.000%	0	0.000%	1	0.002%	0	0.000%

(continued)

MedDRA Preferred Terms	Sub-search	Search 3.1	Search 3.2	Compound 1		Compound 2		Compound 3		Compound 4	
				N	%	N	%	N	%	N	%
Hepatic enzyme increased	2.1	Y		58	1.352%	205	0.829%	96	0.192%	37	0.300%
Hepatic function abnormal	2.1	Y		2	0.047%	141	0.570%	14	0.028%	27	0.219%
Hepatic pain	2.1	Y		1	0.023%	3	0.012%	14	0.028%	0	0.000%
Hepatomegaly	2.1	Y		1	0.023%	23	0.093%	5	0.010%	6	0.049%
Hepatosplenomegaly	2.1	Y		0	0.000%	8	0.032%	3	0.006%	0	0.000%
Hypoalbuminaemia	2.1	Y		1	0.023%	7	0.028%	2	0.004%	0	0.000%
Liver function test abnormal	2.1	Y		10	0.233%	54	0.218%	40	0.080%	14	0.113%
Liver tenderness	2.1	Y		0	0.000%	0	0.000%	1	0.002%	0	0.000%
Urobilin urine present	2.1	Y		0	0.000%	0	0.000%	1	0.002%	0	0.000%
Total number of events in sub-search 2.1	**2.1**			**328**	**7.644%**	**891**	**3.602%**	**380**	**0.761%**	**180**	**1.459%**
Cholestasis	2.2	Y		1	0.023%	51	0.206%	11	0.022%	4	0.032%
Hyperbilirubinaemia	2.2	Y		0	0.000%	29	0.117%	1	0.002%	1	0.008%
Jaundice	2.2	Y		22	0.513%	223	0.902%	34	0.068%	26	0.211%
Jaundice cholestatic	2.2	Y		0	0.000%	30	0.121%	2	0.004%	4	0.032%
Ocular icterus	2.2	Y		2	0.047%	2	0.008%	3	0.006%	0	0.000%
Total number of events in sub-search 2.2	**2.2**			**25**	**0.583%**	**335**	**1.354%**	**51**	**0.102%**	**35**	**0.284%**
Blood thromboplastin abnormal	2.8	Y		1	0.023%	0	0.000%	0	0.000%	0	0.000%
Coagulation factor decreased	2.8	Y		0	0.000%	0	0.000%	1	0.002%	0	0.000%
International normalised ratio abnormal	2.8	Y		0	0.000%	0	0.000%	2	0.004%	0	0.000%
International normalised ratio decreased	2.8	Y		0	0.000%	0	0.000%	6	0.012%	0	0.000%

(continued)

MedDRA Preferred Terms	Sub-search	Search 3.1	Search 3.2	Compound 1		Compound 2		Compound 3		Compound 4	
				N	%	N	%	N	%	N	%
Prothrombin level abnormal	2.8	Y		0	0.000%	0	0.000%	1	0.002%	0	0.000%
Prothrombin level decreased	2.8	Y		0	0.000%	12	0.049%	5	0.010%	1	0.008%
Prothrombin time abnormal	2.8	Y		0	0.000%	0	0.000%	1	0.002%	2	0.016%
Prothrombin time prolonged	2.8	Y		3	0.070%	18	0.073%	13	0.026%	2	0.016%
Prothrombin time ratio decreased	2.8	Y		0	0.000%	1	0.004%	0	0.000%	0	0.000%
Total number of events in sub-search 2.8	**2.8**			**4**	**0.093%**	**31**	**0.125%**	**29**	**0.058%**	**5**	**0.041%**
Number of adverse events and co-manifestations belonging to search 3.1 and/or 3.2 reported with each drug				**390**	**9.089%**	**1679**	**6.788%**	**575**	**1.152%**	**284**	**2.202%**
Total number of adverse events and co-manifestations reported with each drug				**4291**	**100%**	**24735**	**100%**	**49905**	**100%**	**12339**	**100%**

Table 2. Cases identified by searches 3.1 and 3.2.

SMQ Searches	Compound 1		Compound 2		Compound 3		Compound 4	
	N cases	% cases	N cases	% cases	N cases	% cases	N cases	% cases
Search 3.2 (search for severe drug induced liver toxicity)	26	1.52%	394	3.57%	101	0.40%	57	1.00%
Search 3.1* (broad drug induced liver toxicity search)	188	11.03%	702	6.36%	278	1.09%	120	2.11%
Number of cases containing a PT belonging to search 3.1 and/or 3.2	214	12.55%	1106	10.02%	385	1.51%	210	3.70%
Total cases reported with each drug	**1705**	**100.00%**	**11038**	**100.00%**	**25536**	**100.00%**	**5675**	**100.00%**

APPENDIX

Tabulation of Preferred Terms used

Search 1

All terms of searches 2.1 to 2.11

Search 2

Sub-search 2.1

5'nucleotidase increased
Alanine aminotransferase abnormal
Alanine aminotransferase increased
Ammonia abnormal
Ammonia increased
Ascites
Aspartate aminotransferase abnormal
Aspartate aminotransferase increased

Bile output abnormal
Bile output decreased
Bilirubin conjugated increased
Biopsy liver abnormal
Blood alkaline phosphatase abnormal
Blood alkaline phosphatase increased
Blood bilirubin abnormal
Blood bilirubin increased
Blood bilirubin unconjugated increased
Blood cholinesterase abnormal
Blood cholinesterase decreased
Bromosulphthalein test abnormal

Caput medusae

Foetor hepaticus

Galactose elimination capacity test abnormal
Galactose elimination capacity test decreased
Gamma-glutamyltransferase abnormal
Gamma-glutamyltransferase increased
Guanase increased

Haemorrhagic ascites
Hepaplastin abnormal
Hepaplastin decreased
Hepatic congestion
Hepatic enzyme abnormal
Hepatic enzyme decreased
Hepatic enzyme increased
Hepatic function abnormal
Hepatic mass
Hepatic pain
Hepatomegaly
Hepatosplenomegaly
Hyperbilirubinaemia
Hyperammonaemia
Hypercholia
Hypoalbuminaemia

Kayser-Fleischer ring

Leucine aminopeptidase increased
Liver function test abnormal
Liver induration
Liver palpable subcostal
Liver scan abnormal
Liver tenderness

Oedema due to hepatic disease

Perihepatic discomfort

Retinol binding protein decreased

Transaminases abnormal
Transaminases increased

Ultrasound liver abnormal
Urine bilirubin increased
Urobilin urine present

X-ray hepatobiliary abnormal

Sub-search 2.2

Bilirubin excretion disorder

Cholaemia
Cholestasis

Hepatitis cholestatic
Hyperbilirubinaemia

Icterus index increased

Jaundice
Jaundice cholestatic
Jaundice hepatocellular

Ocular icterus

Sub-search 2.3

Autoimmune hepatitis

Chronic hepatitis
Cytolytic hepatitis

Hepatitis
Hepatitis acute
Hepatitis cholestatic
Hepatitis chronic active
Hepatitis chronic persistent
Hepatitis fulminant

Hepatitis granulomatous
Hepatitis toxic

Ischaemic hepatitis

Non-alcoholic steatohepatitis

Radiation hepatitis

Sub-search 2.4

Hepatic cancer metastatic
Hepatic cancer stage I
Hepatic cancer stage II
Hepatic cancer stage III
Hepatic cancer stage IV
Hepatic neoplasm
Hepatic neoplasm malignant
Hepatic neoplasm malignant non-resectable
Hepatic neoplasm malignant recurrent
Hepatic neoplasm malignant resectable
Hepatobiliary carcinoma in situ
Hepatobiliary neoplasm
Hepatoblastoma
Hepatoblastoma recurrent

Liver carcinoma ruptured

Malignant hepatobiliary neoplasm
Mixed hepatocellular cholangiocarcinoma

Sub-search 2.5

Benign hepatic neoplasm

Focal nodular hyperplasia

Haemangioma of liver
Hepatic adenoma
Hepatic cyst
Hepatic cyst ruptured
Hepatic haemangioma rupture

Sub-search 2.6
Ascites
Asterixis

Biliary cirrhosis
Biliary cirrhosis primary
Biliary fibrosis

Coma hepatic

Hepatectomy
Hepatic atrophy
Hepatic cirrhosis
Hepatic encephalopathy
Hepatic failure
Hepatic fibrosis
Hepatic lesion
Hepatic necrosis
Hepatic steatosis
Hepatobiliary disease
Hepatocellular damage
Hepatocellular foamy cell syndrome
Hepatopulmonary syndrome
Hepatorenal failure
Hepatorenal syndrome
Hepatotoxicity

Liver and small intestine transplant
Liver disorder
Liver operation
Liver transplant
Lupoid hepatic cirrhosis

Nodular regenerative hyperplasia
Non-alcoholic steatohepatitis

Oedema due to hepatic disease
Oesophageal varices haemorrhage

Portal hypertension

Portal triaditis

Renal and liver transplant
Reye's syndrome

Spider naevus

Varices oesophageal

Sub-search 2.7

Accessory liver lobe
Alagille syndrome

Cerebrohepatorenal syndrome
Congenital absence of bile ducts
Congenital cystic disease of liver
Congenital hepatic fibrosis
Congenital hepatobiliary anomaly
Congenital hepatomegaly

Dilatation intrahepatic duct congenital

Hepatitis neonatal
Hepatocellular damage neonatal
Hepato-lenticular degeneration
Hepatosplenomegaly neonatal
Hereditary haemochromatosis
Hyperbilirubinaemia neonatal

Jaundice neonatal

Kernicterus

Neonatal cholestasis
Neonatal hepatomegaly

Polycystic liver disease
Porphyria acute
Porphyria non-acute
Pseudoporphyria

Sub-search 2.8

Antithrombin III decreased

Blood fibrinogen abnormal
Blood fibrinogen decreased
Blood thrombin abnormal
Blood thrombin decreased
Blood thromboplastin abnormal
Blood thromboplastin decreased

Coagulation factor decreased
Coagulation factor IX level abnormal
Coagulation factor IX level decreased
Coagulation factor V level abnormal
Coagulation factor V level decreased
Coagulation factor VII level abnormal
Coagulation factor VII level decreased
Coagulation factor X level abnormal
Coagulation factor X level decreased

International normalised ratio abnormal
International normalised ratio decreased

Protein C decreased
Protein S abnormal
Protein S decreased
Prothrombin level abnormal
Prothrombin level decreased
Prothrombin time abnormal
Prothrombin time prolonged
Prothrombin time ratio abnormal
Prothrombin time ratio decreased

Thrombin time abnormal
Thrombin time prolonged

Sub-search 2.9

Adenoviral hepatitis
Amoebic liver abscess

Anti-HBc antibody positive
Anti-HBe antibody positive
Anti-HBc IgM antibody positive
Anti-HBs antibody positive

Congenital hepatitis B infection
Cytomegalovirus hepatitis

Gianotti-Crosti syndrome

Hepatic candidiasis
Hepatic cyst infection
Hepatic echinococciasis
Hepatic infection
Hepatitis A
Hepatitis A antibody abnormal
Hepatitis A antibody positive
Hepatitis A antigen positive
Hepatitis A positive
Hepatitis B
Hepatitis B antibody abnormal
Hepatitis B antibody positive
Hepatitis B core antigen positive
Hepatitis B DNA assay positive
Hepatitis B positive
Hepatitis B surface antigen positive
Hepatitis B e antigen positive
Hepatitis C
Hepatitis C antibody positive
Hepatitis C positive
Hepatitis C RNA positive
Hepatitis D
Hepatitis D antibody positive
Hepatitis D antigen positive
Hepatitis D RNA positive
Hepatitis E
Hepatitis E antibody abnormal
Hepatitis E antibody positive
Hepatitis E antigen positive
Hepatitis F

Hepatitis G
Hepatitis H
Hepatitis infectious
Hepatitis infectious mononucleosis
Hepatitis mumps
Hepatitis non-A non-B
Hepatitis non-A non-B non-C
Hepatitis post transfusion
Hepatitis syphilitic
Hepatitis toxoplasmal
Hepatitis viral
Hepatobiliary infection
Hepatosplenic candidiasis

Liver abscess

Perihepatitis gonococcal
Portal pyaemia

Schistosomiasis liver

Viral hepatitis carrier

Weil's disease

Sub-search 2.10

Alcoholic liver disease

Cirrhosis alcoholic

Fatty liver alcoholic

Hepatitis alcoholic

Zieve syndrome

Sub-search 2.11

Acute fatty liver of pregnancy

Cholestasis of pregnancy

Search 3

Sub-search 3.1

All Terms of Searches 2.1 to 2.6 and 2.8

Sub-search 3.2

All Terms of Searches 2.3 to 2.6

MEMBERS AND PARTICIPANTS OF THE WORKING GROUP

The CIOMS Working Group on Standardised MedDRA Queries (SMQs) met six times from September 2002 until May 2004. Two planning meetings, one in October 2001 in Basel and one in May 2002 in Frankfurt, preceded the establishment of the Working Group in June 2002.

Listed below, followed by a chronology of the work undertaken, are the names of the senior scientists from drug regulatory authorities, WHO, pharmaceutical companies and CIOMS who have participated in all or part of the meetings or otherwise in the project as at August 2004.

Walter Aellig, Novartis	Katja Kusche, Roche
Silvia Bader-Weder, Roche	Magnus Lerch, Schering AG
Cecilia Biriell, WHO-UMC	Sabine Luik, Boehringer-Ingelheim
Mariette Boerstoel, Organon	Kerri MacKay, TGA/Australia
Elliot Brown, Elliot Brown Consulting*	Arthur Meiners, Johnson & Johnson
Mary Couper, WHO	Christiane Michel, Novartis
Isolde Crusius, Boehringer-Ingelheim	Constantin Mirea, Boehringer-Ingelheim
Morell David, MHRA/UK	Odette Morin, ICH/IFPMA
Vikram Dev, AstraZeneca	Patricia Mozzicato, MedDRA/MSSO
Agostino Faggiotto, Pharmacia	Jugo Nermin, Pharmacia
Paul Fallot, Schering-Plough	Norbert Paeschke, BfArM/Germany
Ann Gaines, FDA/USA	Christine Peric, Aventis
Stewart Geary, Eisai	Eva-Beate Rump, MedDRA/MSSO
William W. Gregory, Pfizer	Christina Reith, Roche
Gregory G. Gribko, Pfizer	Yasuo Sakurai, SPJ/Japan
Juhana E. Idänpään-Heikkilä, CIOMS	Marina Sharayeva, Pharma-Center/Ukraine
Kerstin Jansson, MPA/Sweden	Melissa Truffa, FDA/USA
Judith Jones, Degge Group	Panos Tsintis, EMEA/London
Jean Kilgour-Christie, Lilly	Jan Venulet , CIOMS
Chie Kojima, MHLW/Japan	Billy Wilson, Health Canada
Jürgen Köster, Boehringer-Ingelheim	Christina Winter, GSK
Gerhard Kremer, Boehringer-Ingelheim	Hideto Yokoi, NIHS/Japan
Gottfried Kreutz, BfArM/Germany	Tiziana Zaccheo, Pharmacia

* Resigned December 2003

In 2002, CIOMS collected from the regulatory authorities and pharmaceutical companies terms which were considered to be of the highest priority. This produced some 95 terms from which the Working Group selected the first candidate terms to be addressed.

Drafting of a proposal for a SMQ was assigned to a subgroup composed of senior scientists from both regulators and pharmaceutical companies. The candidate SMQ was subsequently considered by the WG during 3-4 meetings and was tested in the databases of both regulators and pharmaceutical companies and the results were fed back to the WG.

The entire process is described in detail in this publication (see the chapter "Overview of Development Concepts Proposed by the Working Group").

By May 2004, the Working Group had met in September 2002 in Basel, January 2003 at EMEA in London, May 2003 at BfArM in Bonn, October 2003 at MHRA in London, February 2004 at IFPMA & WHO in Geneva, and May 2004 at MPA in Uppsala, Sweden.